Be Good to Your Gut

Be Good to Your Gut

Recipes and Tips for People with Digestive Problems

Pat Baird, M.A.,R.D.

Blackwell
Healthcare

Blackwell Science

Editorial offices:

238 Main Street, Cambridge, Massachusetts 02142, USA
Osney Mead, Oxford OX2 0EL, England
25 John Street, London WC1N 2BL, England
23 Ainslie Place, Edinburgh EH3 6AJ, Scotland
54 University Street, Carlton, Victoria 3053, Australia
Arnette Blackwell SA, 1 rue de Lille, 75007 Paris, France
Blackwell Wissenschafts-Verlag GmbH
   Kurfürstendamm 57, 10707 Berlin, Germany
   Feldgasse 13, A-1238 Vienna, Austria

Distributors:

North America
Blackwell Science, Inc.
238 Main Street
Cambridge, Massachusetts 02142
(Telephone orders: 800-215-1000 or 617-876-7000)

Australia
Blackwell Science Pty Ltd
54 University Street
Carlton, Victoria 3053
(Telephone orders: 03-347-0300)

Outside North America and Australia
Blackwell Science, Ltd.
c/o Marston Book Services, Ltd.
P.O. Box 87
Oxford OX2 0DT
England
(Telephone orders: 44-1865-791155)

Acquisitions: William Gibson
Production: Kathleen Grimes
Design, illustrations, and cover photo by Meral Dabcovich,
Visual Perspectives, Brookline, MA

CONTENTS

ACKNOWLEDGMENTS

There's never really a single author of a book. The finished product is always the result of the efforts of many people. I was favored with the talent and support of some of the best all along the way. Let me say "thanks" to all of you.

Bill Gibson and everyone at Blackwell Science, Inc. were enthusiastic from the start. They were eager to help, and were committed at every phase of development, production, and promotion. Julie McQuain is a publicist par excellence. Alice Martell, my agent, is the dream of every author. Her personal care and follow-up brought things along and made the idea a reality.

Rosemary McCoy was invaluable with her help on the recipes and, as always, proved to be a dear and dedicated friend. Lorna Sass is always at my side as a friend and as a professional resource. Her support is ever-present and ever-appreciated. Suzanne Speranza is the manuscript organizer/typist of the century. My books and other projects are always a joy when guided by her watchful eye; this book is just one example of her skills and talent. As always Helen Berman remains my trusted ally. Her strong support and unyielding faith are always there and I treasure them dearly.

Likewise, my sister Rita is a champion of my cause and always ready to help with an idea, a thought, a word, whatever...

No one was more instrumental in the completion of this book than Kathy Leonard. She gave me strength and insight—and lots of her precious time—at a time that was most difficult for me. No words will ever suffice that give Kathy the appreciation of her rare and precious gifts to me.

Other colleagues and friends were a great help from start to finish; they gave me a lot of insight in terms of design and content of the book, and in reading some of the early chapter drafts. Many thanks to Margo Alexander, R.D., Barbara Baron, M.S., R.D., Arnold Berliner, Carol Cappelletti, Peter Cayan, R.D., Marilyn Charwat, Johanna Dwyer, D.Sc., R.D., Michelle Fairchild, M.S., R.D., Deborah Ford Flanel, M.S., R.D., Meghan Flynn, M.S., R.D., Linda Funk, Janet Gibbons, R.D., Judith Gilbride, Ph.D., R.D., Devon Graham, Jean Haggerty, Joann Heppes, M.S., R.D., Shari Kaplan, Julie O'Sullivan-Maillet, Ph.D., R.D., Tom McCann, R.D., Louise Merriman, M.S., R.D., Dennis Savaiano, Ph.D., Margaret Simko, Ph.D., R.D., Annette Warpeha, M.S., R.D.

Be Good to Your Gut

INTRODUCTION

You know the feeling. An hour or so after a meal, something is "burning" behind your breastbone and heading toward your throat. Or to take another example: Before you finish eating, you ache from a cramping pain in the lower abdomen and don't feel better until you've had a bowel movement. You may feel constipated for a few days, and then just as suddenly it's diarrhea from which you're suffering. Or consider a third instance: You can taste the food you'd eaten several days before. Like millions of Americans, your gut is out of order.

The term *gut* generally refers to the alimentary canal: the long muscular tube down which the food we eat gets ground into smaller and smaller particles, is broken down chemically into molecules usable by the body's cells, and finally is either absorbed into the bloodstream or eliminated from the body. Other names for the gut are the digestive tract and gastrointestinal (GI) tract.

The process of digestion, which is what is happening to food in the alimentary canal,

1

involves a complex series of events. For example, different organs produce substances called enzymes which chemically break down food. There is the closely knit network of nerves, muscles, and "messenger chemicals" (neurotransmitters) that work to transport the ingested food through the system—as well as to mix the food with the enzymes and digestive juices.

Not surprisingly, when something goes wrong somewhere in this complex system, we can feel pretty out of sorts in the different ways described above. For some people, such symptoms may require no more than occasionally taking an over-the-counter medication.

However, when GI complaints persist and increase in intensity or frequency, the situation changes. People may now be unable to carry on with their normal daily activities. They soon worry that the increasingly distressing problem may be a sign of a very serious disease, like an ulcer or a heart attack.

Hopefully, in your case, some of the information in this book will prevent that from happening. For those of you who already have had a persistent GI problem, take heart. Many cases of serious disorders respond well to treatment, and often the disorder can be prevented from returning. But before we talk about some of the solutions, let's take a quick, selective glance at how

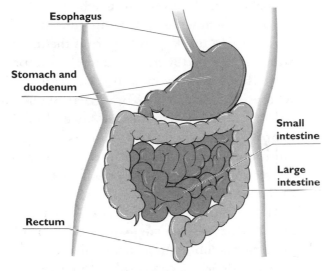

THE GASTROINTESTINAL TRACT

the gut works.

The digestive tract spans the mouth, esophagus, stomach, and small and large intestines (see Figure). In addition, the salivary glands, liver, and pancreas produce enzymes that help to metabolize protein, starches, sugars, and fat. These secretions combine with similar enzymes produced by glands in the stomach and intestinal walls.

Digestion begins in the mouth with the chewing of food and the action of saliva, which contains enzymes that begin to change some of the food starches into sugar. Food is then swallowed and enters the esophagus. From there, wave-like muscular contractions—called peristalsis—quickly propel the food into the stomach.

Rings of muscle at various junctures in the digestive tract open to permit the ingested food to pass downward, and close to prevent that mass from being pushed back where it came from. To a great extent, a defective muscle band at the far end of the esophagus called the lower esophageal sphincter is responsible for the onset of heartburn, which was described at the start of this introduction.

If the pancreas produces insufficient amounts of the enzyme insulin, or no insulin at all, a person cannot metabolize carbohydrates properly. The result is diabetes mellitus. A problem in diabetics resulting from GI nerve damage is called gastroparesis. The stomach muscles are slow to push the partially digested food into the small intestine, and that's the reason diabetics often feel full after eating only small portions of a meal. It's also why they say they can taste food eaten days earlier.

Various GI symptoms are thought to be due to lactose intolerance, or an inability to break down a sugar found in milk and dairy products. On the basis of that assumption, people are frequently told to restrict or eliminate their consumption of dairy products. If this has been the case for you, or if you suspect that you have a problem with lactose, be sure to read "A New Look at Lactose." This chapter takes a look at lactose in a practical way that will be useful for the majority of people with such concerns.

Thus, within the complexity of the digestive process, some common elements have been identified. Heartburn and gastroparesis are examples of motility disorders, in which there is a problem with either muscular activity in the digestive tract or the nerves regulating that activity. Diabetes mellitus and lactose intolerance are examples of problems arising from the absence or deficiency of an enzyme necessary for complete digestion. Some other GI problems—constipation, irritable bowel syndrome and indigestion—will also be covered in separate chapters.

"Be good to your gut" suggests a reciprocal relationship between how you treat your body—specifically, your digestive system—and how you feel. The information throughout this book will give you a great deal of insight into how much of that relationship is within your control. The body is an amazing machine. Like a car, it performs better when you take good care of it and put the right fuel into the tank. In many cases, when you are good to your gut, it will be good to you.

The key components of caring for your digestive system include diet, exercise, and stress management. This book will focus mainly on diet. However, the cornerstone messages of good nutrition—variety, moderation, and balance—are the same for other areas of your life. These "guideposts" also are the essence of successful weight management and overall good health.

With regard to diet, it is helpful to understand that *variety* means choosing a wide array of foods from each of the food groups on a daily basis. *Moderation* and *balance* suggest commonsense portions in the meals or snacks that are eaten. There are many guides for determining the right size of portions, from package labels to the recommendations of the U.S.D.A. Food Guide Pyramid. They indicate very specific amounts for virtually every food. Though some of these portions (or servings) seem small, most people recognize that an 18-ounce steak or a pint of ice cream really is not "a serving."

These messages of good nutrition—variety, moderation, and balance—are also useful to anyone with a GI problem. As you read the chapters, you'll see that some ailments may have more specific guidelines than others, but often the advice is similar. For example, you will be encouraged to reduce your intake of foods high in fat and concentrate more on other foods. This recommendation is equally applicable in heartburn, gastroparesis, and irritable bowel syndrome.

So now you can see that much of your own comfort and well-being is within your control. Depending on the severity of your symptom, a good diet may take you a long way towards good health. In some instances you may need special medication. The following chapters should provide you with the information to get you started in the right direction. The final chapter provides a list of resource organizations and recommends some books for further reading. These should help you be good to your gut for a long time.

GUIDELINES FOR EVERYONE

Stress, tension, diet, and poor eating habits all contribute to gastrointestinal problems. There are a few tips that can be helpful to anyone plagued with those problems. Although the following chapters deal with specific GI disorders, there are some general considerations that can be useful in practically all cases.

Keep a Food Diary. That means writing down everything you eat throughout the day. It is most beneficial if you can make notes as close to the time that you eat as possible. To do that, consider carrying a small spiral notebook in your pocket or purse. A few small index cards will also do the trick. In addition to writing down what you ate, also include how much you ate, what time it was, whom you were with, how you were feeling, and what the ingredients in the foods and beverages were (especially if you're trying to uncover an irritant food or spice). A food diary is probably your best resource for uncovering a specific problem.

It can also provide the information to solve that problem.

Get to Know Gas-Producing Foods. Many foods such as beans and cruciferous vegetables, like cauliflower and broccoli, commonly produce gas in a lot of people. Gas is very uncomfortable as well as being an embarrassing problem. However, those nutritious foods provide a variety of vitamins and minerals, and they are a good source of fiber. So try not to eliminate them unless it's absolutely essential. Instead, experiment with different foods, and carefully observe (using the food diary) what, if any, reaction you have.

Even if you have already abandoned some of these, you might find you *can* eat them if you do so in smaller amounts. Often it is large portions which cause distress. Or, perhaps you can learn new ways to prepare these foods which reduce the gas (some ideas for preparing dried beans, for instance, are in the "Checklist" on page 11). A list of some of the common gas-producing foods is provided at the end of this chapter, and in the irritable bowel syndrome chapter.

Dairy foods can often be enjoyed even if you think you are lactose intolerant. Here too, it is the *amount* of food, rather than the particular food, that creates the problem for many people. A large dish of ice cream, for example, or a bowl of cereal with lots of milk first thing in the morning produces discomfort in some folks. But an ounce or two of cheese, or some cottage cheese in a casserole, or a spoonful of grated cheese over pasta is really quite tolerable for the majority of people. Likewise, a small glass of milk with a few crackers or a piece of angel food cake is also tolerable even though milk may have been on the "eliminate" list. Dairy foods are important to people of all ages. Overall, these foods provide lots of good nutrition: vitamins, minerals, protein, and carbohydrate. The large selection of low-fat and fat-free products now available is an added bonus. They can help everyone get their quota of these important foods each day, without having too much fat.

If you truly are lactose intolerant, you may be able to tolerate yogurt and other cultured products like aged cheese or buttermilk. The section on lactose (page 221) gives you more information on products which can help you enjoy a wider variety of foods. It may also help you determine whether you are truly lactose intolerant.

CHECKLIST

Following some very simple suggestions often reduces the number of digestive problems you experience. Look at the
list below, and see if you have any lifestyle
habits that could be adding to your discomfort. If so, these pointers may help
you turn them around, and provide some
quick relief.

1. Eat Slowly.

2. Chew food thoroughly.

3. Keep portions small to moderate,
and avoid overeating.

4. Avoid constipation. Eat fiber, drink
water, and allow yourself time to go
to the bathroom.

5. Exercise regularly.

6. Limit fluids, especially carbonated
drinks, with meals.

7. Sip, rather than gulp, carbonated
drinks when you do drink them.

8. Avoid swallowing air. For some people this is a nervous habit or the
result of stress. Chewing gum, suck-
ing on hard candies, smoking, exces-

sive salivation (often due to poor-fitting dentures), and drinking from straws and bottles encourages air to be swallowed and gas to form.

9. Soak dried beans overnight; drain and cover with fresh water to cook. Or use a quick presoak if desired. Cover beans with water. Bring to a boil and cook for 2 minutes. Remove from heat; let stand for 1 hour. Drain, and cover with fresh water to cook.

10. Add yogurt with live-active cultures to recipes with gas-producing foods, or have some with your meal. Acidophilus bacteria in yogurt slows down gas production for some people, and helps to digest food more easily.

11. Try BEANO, a new product from the folks who developed Lactaid. It contains a digestive enzyme that helps to digest beans and legumes.

SPICES

Spices add flavor and enhance the taste of many foods. When you're trying to cut down on fat that can be very helpful. Though fat adds to the taste and satisfaction of food, unfortunately, it also adds a lot of calories. For many Americans who are overweight, that's a big consideration. In addition, fat also contributes to many gastrointestinal problems.

So, lower-fat diets have several benefits. Not only can they be helpful for weight loss, they also can be especially important in alleviating some GI symptoms. The dilemma is that low-fat meals tend to lose flavor when they lose fat. Using a variety of herbs and spices is a good way to reduce some of the fat in recipes and still keep the enjoyment in meals.

A number of people with gastrointestinal problems gravitate—or are counselled—toward a bland and spice-free menu. What a mistake! That's not always necessary, and besides, eating bland, dull food is boring. Eventually people on such a program will be tempted to "cheat" or binge. And then the results are definitely painful.

Instead of trying a bland diet, take another look at spices. In many cases, a more individualized approach that includes herbs and spices, can be the solution. You may already be certain that some of these ingredients are definite irritants for you. By all means, then, avoid them.

But don't cross everything off the list. Try some of the acceptable spices on page 15 the next time you're cooking, and see which you tolerate better. You'll probably discover that you can put flavor and pleasure back into your meals. You might even eat less because you're more satisfied. Eating less will help you to lose weight, feel better, and soothe some of your GI distress.

Remember that not all spices are irritating to the stomach. Garlic, black pepper, chili pepper, chili powder, curry powder, cloves, and nutmeg seem to give people the most problems. On the other hand, rosemary, basil, thyme, paprika, caraway seed, cinnamon, allspice, and mace are less likely to aggravate the GI tract.

Sometimes eating any spicy food on an empty stomach can cause distress, especially in people with heartburn or irritable bowel syndrome. Something as simple as having a few crackers, a slice of bread, or a roll before eating helps to reduce the harsh reaction. Adjustments such as these allow a wider variety of foods to be enjoyed. Experiment a little and see what works for

14

you. Just be sure to write down the details as you go along. That way you can "track" different spices and situations and see what's best for you.

Here is a list of some common herbs, spices, and foods for you to review. Some are generally pretty "safe" for GI patients, while others are commonly aggravating. There is also a list of several items which generally irritate the esophagus.

Remember, these lists are only meant to be guides. Some of these items will not be a problem for many people, while others, not listed here, are definitely hazards.

Acceptable Spices:

dill	cumin
basil	cilantro
rosemary	chervil
thyme	sage

Troublesome Spices:

pepper	chili powder
garlic	nutmeg
mint	mustard seeds
cloves	

Esophageal Irritants:

tomatoes	citrus fruits & juices: orange, lemon, lime, grapefruit

continued...

Gas Producing Foods:

Fruits:

Apples (raw)
Apple juice
Avocado
Bananas
Cantaloupe
Honeydew
Grapes
Raisins
Watermelon

Misc.:

Carbonated
  beverages
Chewing gum
Hard candy
Nuts
Mannitol and
  Sorbitol —
  synthetic
  sweeteners
Fats and high fat
  foods
Rich sauces,
  gravies

Vegetables:

Beans (kidney, lima, navy)
Broccoli
Brussels sprouts
Cabbage
Cauliflower
Corn
Cucumbers
Leeks
Onions
Split peas
Lentils
Peppers, green
Radishes
Scallions
Shallots
Soybeans

Cereals and Grains:

Bran Cereals
Excessive quantities of wheat products

BASIC RECIPES

Here are a few recipes that are also used as part of recipes in other sections of the book. They are good "staple" items which can be enjoyed by virtually everyone.

Vegetable Stock

Mushroom Stock

Fluffy Rice

Brown Rice

Creamy Yogurt Sauce

Vegetable Stock

Makes about 2 quarts

Here is a lovely stock that makes a great stand-in for canned chicken broth. It freezes beautifully so there's no reason not to have some on hand at all times. It's especially nice for making risotto or just basic rice (page 22).

1 tablespoon olive oil

1 large onion, coarsely chopped, *optional*

2 medium carrots, *scrubbed and sliced*

2 medium parsnips, *scrubbed and sliced*

2 celery ribs, *with leaves, sliced*

1 medium zucchini, *(about 8 ounces), sliced*

6 sprigs parsley

1 teaspoon chopped fresh thyme *or* *1/2 teaspoon dried*

2 bay leaves

4 quarts water

Salt & freshly ground black pepper to taste

In a large stock pot or Dutch oven heat the oil over high heat. Add the onions (if using), carrots, parsnips, and celery. Cook for 3 minutes. Add the remaining ingredients, except the salt, and pepper.

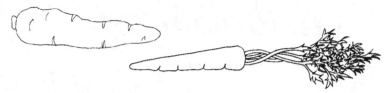

Reduce the heat to low. Cover partially, and cook for about 1 hour. Remove cover, and simmer about 30 minutes longer. Strain the stock into a bowl, gently pressing the liquid out of the vegetables with the back of a spoon. Let cool; add salt and pepper to taste. Store in covered containers, or freeze for later use.

TASTE TIP:

Use 1 teaspoon onion powder if you're very sensitive to onion, and omit pepper if necessary. A pinch of nutmeg and a pinch of crushed red pepper flakes are nice additions too, as tolerated.

NUTRITION VALUES PER 1-CUP SERVING
Calories 18.1
Fat 1.7g
Cholesterol 0.0mg
Sodium 38.9mg
Protein 0.19g
Carbohydrates .74g
Fiber 0.1g

Mushroom Stock

Makes about 2 quarts

This stock is so rich and delicious that you can merely add some cooked rice or pasta and some vegetables for a lovely light meal. It's also very satisfying on its own as a soothing consommé. Try it in the mushroom risotto (page 144) for a truly divine creation.

1 tablespoon vegetable oil

2 medium leeks, *(white part only), thoroughly washed and thinly sliced*

2 cloves garlic, *chopped, optional*

3/4 pound fresh white mushrooms, *sliced*

1 1/2 ounces dried shitake mushrooms, *broken into pieces*

4 sprigs parsley

1/2 teaspoon dried sage leaves

5 allspice berries

9 cups water

Salt and freshly ground black pepper to taste

In a stock pot or Dutch oven heat the oil over high heat. Add the leeks, garlic (if using), and fresh mushrooms, and cook for 2 minutes. Add the remaining ingredients, except the salt and pepper. Reduce heat to low. Cover partially, and cook for about 45 minutes.

Strain the stock into a bowl, gently pressing the liquid out of the vegetables with the back of a spoon. Let cool; add salt and pepper to taste. Store in covered containers, or freeze for later use.

TASTE TIP:

Use 1/2 teaspoon garlic powder for garlic cloves if desired; omit pepper if necessary.

NUTRITION VALUES PER 1-CUP SERVING
Calories 16.4
Fat 1.7g
Cholesterol 0.0mg
Sodium 32.0mg
Protein 0.0g
Carbohydrates 0.3g
Fiber 0.0g

Fluffy Rice

Makes about 4 servings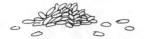

Always check the package directions, as some types of rice may vary the amount of liquid a bit. But for the most part, here's a reliable version.

1 cup regular white rice

2 cups liquid *(water, broth, or juice)*

2 teaspoons butter *or* vegetable oil, *optional*

1/2 teaspoon salt

In a medium saucepan combine all the ingredients. Bring to a boil, and stir. Reduce heat to low. Cover, and simmer for about 15 minutes, or until the rice is cooked, and most of the liquid is absorbed. Fluff with a fork and serve, or cool and freeze for later use.

Microwave Method:

In a medium microwavable casserole combine all the ingredients. Cover, and microwave on HIGH for 5 minutes, or until boiling. Reduce setting to MEDIUM, and cook 15 minutes longer, or until the rice is cooked and most of the liquid is absorbed.

Conventional Oven:

This is especially handy when other foods are baking.

Preheat oven to 350°F.

Use boiling liquid to start. Then combine all the ingredients in a 1 1/2-quart casserole dish. Cover tightly, and bake for about 25 minutes, or until the rice is cooked and most of the liquid is absorbed.

Electric Rice Cookers:

These are very practical appliances to own — especially if you're a fan of rice. The automatic ones will keep rice warm and fluffy all day, and can be programmed to cook the rice at a certain time even if you're not home.

Combine all ingredients, using 1/4 to 1/2 cup less water than usual. See manufacturers' directions for setting instructions.

NUTRITION VALUES PER SERVING
Calories 189.5
Fat 2.3g
Cholesterol 5.5mg
Sodium 292.8mg
Protein 3.2g
Carbohydrates 37.8g
Fiber 0.2g

Brown Rice

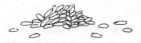

Extra time is needed to cook brown rice. It has a bit more fiber than white rice, but not a significant amount. Brown rice does have a deeper, nutty taste and a coarser texture than white rice. That can offer some benefits in certain recipes.

1 cup brown rice

2 1/4 cups liquid *(water, broth, or juice)*

2 teaspoons butter *or* vegetable oil, *optional*

3/4 teaspoon salt

In a medium saucepan combine all the ingredients. Bring to a boil, and stir. Reduce heat to low. Cover, and simmer for about 45 minutes, or until the rice is cooked and most of the liquid is absorbed. Fluff with a fork and serve or cool and freeze for later use.

Microwave Method:

In a medium microwavable casserole combine all ingredients. Cover, and microwave on HIGH for 5 minutes, or until boiling. Reduce setting to MEDIUM, and cook 45 minutes longer, or until the rice is cooked and most of the liquid is absorbed.

Conventional Oven:

Preheat oven to 350°F.

Use boiling liquid to start. Then combine all the ingredients in a 1 1/2-quart casserole dish Cover tightly, and bake for about 1 hour, or until the rice is cooked and most of the liquid is absorbed.

NUTRITION VALUES PER SERVING
Calories 224.9
Fat 3.3g
Cholesterol 5.5mg
Sodium 434.4mg
Protein 5.4g
Carbohydrates 46.2g
Fiber 2.7g

Creamy Yogurt Sauce

Makes about 1 cup

Try this versatile sauce over fresh berries, fresh or canned sliced fruits, fat-free pound cake, or angel food cake. It adds a nice touch to desserts without adding fat, and it's bound to please every member of the family.

1 cup nonfat plain yogurt

1 tablespoon honey

2 teaspoons lemon juice

1/2 teaspoon vanilla extract

In a small bowl whisk together all the ingredients. Cover, and refrigerate until ready to serve.

TASTE TIP:

Use any variety of juice to vary the taste a bit. The small amount should not be an irritant, but you may omit it without any great flavor loss. Use a little more honey instead.

NUTRITION VALUES PER 1/4-CUP SERVING
Calories 45.6
Fat 0.0g
Cholesterol 1.0mg
Sodium 43.7mg
Protein 2.3g
Carbohydrates 7.8g
Fiber 0.0g

CONSTIPATION

By any yardstick, constipation is a common problem, affecting about 1 in every 50 people. Even so, it's surprising to discover that this ailment accounts for about 2.5 million visits to physicians annually. And almost 100,000 individuals are hospitalized each year for what are described as constipation-related problems.

With that in mind, it's not surprising to see the number of ads for laxatives aimed at helping to keep us "regular." But what is regular? And what is constipation really? Some people will say their stools are too hard or dry or that they have to strain to move their bowels. Others will note that they have infrequent bowel movements. The definition of constipation for many physicians, and the one used in clinical research, is having fewer than three bowel movements a week.

Nevertheless, individuals can and do vary on what is normal for them. So your bowel movements could be fine if you "go" as often as three times a day, and you don't necessarily have constipation if you go as infrequently as every fifth day. Certainly, the notion that one bowel movement every day is essential is pure fallacy.

Constipation seems to occur in some people more often than in others. Women are more prone than men, especially during pregnancy. Increased pressure on the bowel from the fetus, a decline in gut motility, and less physical activity all contribute to constipation at this time.

People older than 65 also are affected more frequently. Many factors combine to cause constipation: a general slowing down of bodily functions as one ages; poor nutrition, which might come about because of less money to spend on food, loss of a spouse, or lack of family or friends with whom to share meals; not drinking enough fluids; lack of physical activity; or taking certain medications. Other lifestyle factors or habits, in people of all ages, can lead to constipation. Irregular eating and drinking, as well as travel—whether for business or pleasure—are all potential reasons for constipation to occur.

A very common cause of constipation is overuse of laxatives. People who habitually take laxatives eventually become dependent on them. That means laxatives are taken in larger amounts and with greater frequency, until finally the small intestine and colon no longer work on their own and daily laxatives become the norm. This condition is known as a cathartic colon, or "lazy bowel."

Other drugs can also have a constipating effect, including pain relievers, aluminum-containing antacids, and iron supplements. Medications to control high blood pressure, antispasmodic drugs, and antidepressants are other possible "culprits." The list on page 39 gives you a better idea of the classes of drugs that can cause constipation.

Not to be overlooked as a factor in chronic constipation are dramatic changes in the American diet. A century or so ago the average daily consumption of fiber was at least 40 grams. Today the daily average is about 10 grams. When you take a look at what we're eating today--lots of refined foods that contain fat, sugar, and calories, but not much fiber—it's easy to understand why. When the reduction in fiber intake is accompanied by a basically sedentary lifestyle, constipation is often the result.

Finally, when constipation is a chronic problem, it may indicate a serious underlying disease. Irritable bowel syndrome is one of the most common causes of constipation in the United States. Uncoordinated muscular contractions in people with IBS can delay the movement of bowel contents, leading to constipation. Other gastrointestinal disorders—for example, inflammatory bowel disease or hemorrhoids—may produce an obstruction or narrowed passageway, or can cause painful elimination.

In other situations, hormonal distur-
bances, such as an underactive thyroid, can
be the problem. Diabetics frequently suffer
from constipation. Neurologic diseases such
as stroke, multiple sclerosis, and Parkinson's
disease, also are linked to constipation.

The good news is that constipation is not
only treatable, but also preventable. In
many cases, dietary changes are the answer.

What to Do about It

Prevention is the key word when it comes
to constipation. For the most part, a balanced diet with an emphasis on fiber is the
first line of defense. Drinking lots of fluids
and making exercise part of your general
routine also will help you stay regular.

Time is an important consideration that
people often overlook when it comes to preventing constipation. Allowing time to "heed
the call of nature" shouldn't be ignored.
With busy schedules and hectic lifestyles, we
sometimes rush ourselves or even try to postpone going to the bathroom until a more convenient time. Unfortunately, the latter habit
may lead to a loss of our rectal reflexes.

For most people, the morning seems to be
"their time." Perhaps it's drinking hot liquids or stimulants such as caffeine that is
responsible for the urge to go. Whatever
the reason, be sure to allow enough time to

have a full and relaxed movement. If the feeling comes later in the day, give yourself the few minutes it takes at that time for an undisturbed visit to the bathroom.

If you notice any change in bowel habits that persists for several weeks, it's a good idea to see your physician. Sometimes, constipation is related to other conditions. If you think you're already eating a healthy variety of foods and drinking plenty of water, and yet you develop a constipation problem, a checkup is definitely in order.

Diet Natural fiber is readily available in a variety of foods. And let's face it, food is a tastier way of reducing, if not eliminating, constipation than fiber laxatives. So what is fiber? And how much of it should we be eating each day?

Fiber is the part of plant foods we eat that is resistant to normal digestive processes. It is found in vegetables, fruits, whole grains, nuts, and seeds, and not at all in meat, milk, or other dairy products. Also referred to as bulk or roughage, fiber in your diet helps keep you regular. There are other great reasons to boost your daily fiber intake: A high-fiber diet is a treatment for diverticulosis, a disorder in which the bowel wall folds outward and forms small pouches which can trap food and become infected. Fiber also may have a positive role in the management of high cholesterol and diabetes, and it may even reduce the risk of developing certain types of cancer.

Including more fiber in your diet goes way beyond bran cereals and prune juice. But don't overlook these foods—they're a good way to get a head start on your fiber quota first thing in the morning. A high-fiber diet is varied and contains a wide array of foods, including whole-grain breads and cereals, beans, lentils, vegetables, and fruits.

The recommended amount of fiber is about 20 to 35 grams per day. (Dietitians often base fiber requirements on the amount of calories consumed and figure 10 to 13 grams per 1,000 calories.) That is almost double the amount of fiber that most Americans actually consume now.

Knowing the amount of "dietary" fiber in food is more important than knowing about "crude" fiber. The latter is what remains and is measured in the laboratory after acid and alkali digestion. It's really a scientific term that doesn't have much meaning for the general public. Dietary fiber, on the other hand, is determined by laboratory analysis of food and represents the total fiber content of the individual food.

Dietary fiber is classified according to how soluble it is in water. Foods like oat bran, barley, lentils, carrots, plums, apricots, bananas, and pears contain *soluble* fiber. Soluble fibers are sticky and combine with water to form gels. They have a role in the function of the digestive tract, but seem to play a bigger part in reducing blood cholesterol and may reduce insulin needs in some diabetics.

Insoluble fiber is composed largely of cellulose and lignin—the chewy outer parts of seeds or fruit skins, husks, and peels. It is also found in wheat germ, dried peas and beans, cornmeal, millet, and apples. Insoluble fiber, especially wheat bran, is particularly effective in the treatment of chronic constipation. This type of fiber tends to act mainly as a bulking agent; that is, it absorbs large amounts of water and creates a soft, bulky stool. Stool weight is also increased, and the combined effect is to reduce the time it takes for digested food to move through the digestive tract. So you can see how it can be effective in the treatment of constipation. Regulating intestinal "transit time" means that, in some cases, fiber also can be effective in the treatment of diarrhea. The chart on page 40 is a handy reference for distinguishing between insoluble and soluble fiber.

When you start on your fiber program, a few suggestions are in order. First, do it slowly. Fiber can produce gas and bloating, especially in the beginning. Try to spread your fiber intake throughout the day. Don't just load up on a big bowl of bran and fruit in the morning.

Second, drink lots of water. Remember

that fiber works because of its ability to hold water. If there's not enough water around in your gut, the fiber will literally get stuck and produce severe constipation. A minimum of eight glasses of water a day is essential to keep that fiber moving along.

Other Factors   A regular exercise program also helps bowel regularity. It keeps the blood circulating and all systems "go." Exercise also contributes to overall good health and to a positive mental outlook, so the benefits of physical activity are numerous.

Biofeedback training may be of benefit. Sometimes excessive tension or inappropriate constriction of muscles contributes to constipation. There is evidence that after a few biofeedback sessions patients can learn to substitute normal relaxation of rectal muscles for the tightening or contracting they may have been doing inadvertently.

To be most effective, any changes you adopt should happen gradually. Be patient. It may take a few weeks for your body to adjust. Changes should not be disruptive; that way, there's a better chance they'll become an integral part of your life.

A Word about Laxatives

Laxatives can be used occasionally. But their use really should be a last resort.

Dependence on, or overuse of, laxatives has its own problems. Muscles get lazy when they are artificially stimulated all the time (as with a laxative). Over time, muscle tension is reduced or lost. However, that cycle can be broken. If you are in that predicament, take heart. Reduce laxative use gradually and follow the suggestions below. In a couple of weeks, you should be doing fine on your own. Pregnant women should avoid taking any laxative unless it's recommended by their physicians. Increased consumption of fruits, vegetables, cereals, and grains, along with more water and physical activity, is the best solution during this time.

Several types of laxatives are available and work in a variety of ways. They include fiber, lubricants, emollient laxatives, and stimulant cathartics.

Fiber such as bran or psyllium is a bulk-forming agent. It swells, absorbs water, and helps to move digested foods through the intestinal tract and out of the body. Grandma's favorite standby, mineral oil, is an example of the lubricant type of laxative. However, mineral oil can also interfere with the absorption of calcium and fat-soluble vitamins (A, D, E, and K), so try to avoid it. Emollient laxatives are also known as stool softeners; for the most, part they are not too effective and are not recommended for long-term use. Stimulant cathartics—for example, senna, bisacodyl, and phenolphthalein—are frequently found in over-the-counter preparations. Check the label for ingredients in your brand. These compounds are not recommended for long-term use; yet physicians find that many people become dependent on them. If you think you're overusing stimulant cathartics now, taper them off gradually while you add more water and fiber to your diet.

Other Drugs for Constipation

Improvement in constipation has been reported with some medications. Cisapride (Propulsid®), a promotility drug useful for nighttime heartburn, has been shown to increase bowel movements and reduce laxative use. Misoprostol (Cytotec®), a prostaglandin compound used to treat injuries of the stomach related to NSAID use, is known to cause diarrhea. Naloxone (Narcan®), a treatment for opiate abusers, may produce improvement in some constipated individuals. It should be noted that these drugs are not currently approved by the U.S. Food and Drug Administration (FDA) for use in treating constipation.

Summary

Speak to your physician if constipation is

a serious problem for you. It's particularly important to have this discussion if you are overusing laxatives or think you may be becoming dependent on them.

Finally, keeping a diary can be helpful. Note down when you get the urge to defecate, how much water you're drinking, what you are eating, and how much fiber you're getting. Observing the effects of your behavior will help you find your personal solution to constipation.

Some drugs that can cause constipation

Analgesics (pain relievers)

Antacids (calcium and aluminum)

Anticholinergics

Anticonvulsants

Antidepressants

Antihypertensives

Antiparkinsonian drugs

Diuretics

Iron supplements

MAO inhibitors

Opiates

Psychoactive drugs

Fiber at a Glance

Here's a quick reference chart to show you foods that contain soluble and insoluble fiber. Note that some foods contain both types of fiber. Though you should have some of both kinds each day for your over-all health, it's the insoluble fiber that works best in reducing constipation.

Insoluble	Soluble
Wheat bran	Oat bran
Corn bran	Rice bran
Whole grains (wheatberries, etc.)	Chick peas
	Dried beans
Dried beans (kidney, navy etc.)	Sesame seeds
Canned beans	All fruits and vegetables
Nuts and seeds	especially apples plums, pears, carrots
Most fruits and vegetables especially potatoes, broccoli, parsnips	

Fiber Supplements

No doubt you've seen a number of fiber supplements in the store, ranging from bran tablets to cellulose powders. They can, indeed, be effective in treating constipation. For some individuals, however, they can produce side effects like gas, bloating, nausea, and abdominal discomfort. That's because these products consist of a highly purified form of fiber. As a dietitian it is always a perplexing question for me when people ask my opinion about these products. I'm a firm believer in real food. Though a fiber supplement may do the job, it lacks the variety of nutrients found in food. Because nutrition is a relatively young science, new nutrients and the role they play in maintaining good health probably have yet to be discovered. So choose fruits, vegetables, grains, cereals, beans, and lentils for your sources of fiber. You'll get an array of colors, tastes, and textures, as well as a lot more pleasure from eating wholesome foods along with it.

Quick Tips to Boost Your Fiber Intake

- Stir frozen vegetables into your favorite soup, sauce, or casserole. Broccoli and cauliflower in a tomato sauce, corn in chili, or mixed vegetables into chicken soup are just a few suggestions to get you started.

- Sprinkle some wheat germ over hot cereals, salads, or grain dishes.

- Order brown rice in Chinese restaurants.

- Toss cooked or canned (drained) beans into soups, salads, and pasta dishes.

- Use cooked lentils in rice pilafs, burger and meatloaf mixtures, and pasta sauces.

- Sprinkle frozen (and thawed) peas, broccoli, or corn onto pizza before baking.

- Add fresh and dried fruits to muffin and quick bread recipes.

- Save the pulp from your juicer and add to soups, sauces, and cake recipes.

- Try air-popped popcorn as a snack instead of pretzels or chips.

- Serve drained slices or chunks of canned fruit over cereals, slices of fat-free pound cake, or frozen yogurt.

Beyond Fresh: Fruit and Vegetable Fiber Bonuses

Most people are hooked on the notion that freshly picked fruits and vegetables are

42

the best, and perhaps the only way to get the highest amount of fiber and nutrients. Fortunately, that's just not so. Sure, nothing beats a fresh, juicy peach in the middle of summer, and if you're lucky enough to live close to a farm, or have access to a farmer's market, chances are you're getting a high nutritional value. But it's time for everyone to take another look at canned and frozen fruits and vegetables to find out what they offer.

Variety is the cornerstone of good nutrition. In reality, a combination of canned and frozen fruits and vegetables offers the best and most convenient way to ensure practical, as well as tasty, nutrition. There are literally dozens of items from which to choose, and a variety of forms in which they are packed. It's time to let go of the notion that frozen or canned items are necessarily loaded with fat, sodium, and sugar, or that they are automatically less nutritious than their fresh counterparts. If you have any question just take a look at some labels next time you're in the supermarket to see what's not in a lot of these foods.

Today frozen fruits and vegetables are flash frozen at the peak of freshness within hours of harvest. This process helps to preserve nutrients.

In fact there have been several studies that show that frozen items actually contain as much, or more, nutrient value as raw produce. That's because it may take several days for the fresh food to be packaged and then shipped to the supermarket. Add a few more days of storage time in the refrigerator at home, and more nutrients are lost.

From a practical point of view, frozen and canned items are always ready to go. There's no cleaning, peeling, cutting, and trimming for you to do. Simply open the package or the can and add the contents to your favorite recipe. When using frozen items, I find it particularly helpful to buy them in plastic bags. They defrost faster, and it's easier to measure out a cup or two from a bag than it is to try to separate a solid block.

In terms of fiber content, corn, spinach, and peas rate especially high, as do the cruciferous vegetables such as Brussels sprouts, broccoli, bok choy, cauliflower, and collard greens. The latter are also rich sources of vitamin A. Though each of these vegetables is packaged individually, there are also many interesting frozen vegetable combinations that contain three or four different types of vegetables in the same bag. These make a great addition to pasta or rice for a quick and easy primavera dish, or you can toss them with lettuce for a five-minute salad.

Frozen and canned fruits shouldn't be overlooked either. Frozen berries are a great way to enjoy these summer treats all year long. They can be used for fruit purees to serve over desserts, blended with yogurt for healthy drinks, or tossed into muffin batters. Canned fruits offer good nutrition and good taste. Remember that canned fruits are now packed in natural juices as well as in traditional heavy syrups. Canned pears and peaches are especially high in fiber. You might add canned peaches to a fresh spinach salad, or toss canned pear slices with fresh berries for a stunning dessert.

RECIPES

Double Apricot Shake

Sunny Orange Bran Muffins

Country Vegetable-Bean Soup

Vegetarian Split Pea Soup

Pineapple-Cucumber Salsa

Spinach-Bean Dip

Gingered Chicken

Jerk Pork Tenderloin with Black Beans

Roasted Vegetables and Idaho Potatoes

Yellow Rice with Black Beans and Peas

Cranberry-Yogurt Coffee Cake

Apple-Oatmeal Crisp

Strawberries and Pears with Creamy Yogurt Sauce

Double Apricot Shake

Makes 2 servings

There's more than just fiber in this tasty drink. Yogurt means lots of calcium, and apricots add vitamin A. Wheat germ lends a nutty taste, and a little extra texture also.

1 cup nonfat plain yogurt

1 5 1/4-ounce can apricot nectar

1 4-ounce can apricots, *packed in juice, drained*

2 tablespoons wheat germ

1 tablespoon honey

2 ice cubes, *optional*

Place all the ingredients in a blender. Cover, and blend on high speed until smooth. Serve immediately.

TASTE TIP:

Use any of your favorite fruits: berries, pears, or kiwi are nice choices and good sources of fiber. Substitute orange juice for the apricot nectar as tolerated.

NUTRITION VALUES PER SERVING
Calories 199.4
Fat 0.9g
Cholesterol 7.0mg
Sodium 99.8mg
Protein 7.2g
Carbohydrates 39.7g
Fiber 1.0g

Sunny Orange Bran Muffins

Makes 9 muffins

Orange juice stands in for the milk tradition-
ally used in muffins. So if you're the least bit
lactose sensitive, these are a great way to get
your fiber intake. Feel free to add some
chopped nuts, or sesame or sunflower seeds
(as tolerated) to boost the fiber.

1 cup unprocessed bran flakes

2/3 cup whole-wheat flour

2/3 cup all-purpose flour

1/3 cup sugar

1 tablespoon baking powder

**1/2 teaspoon *each* ground cinnamon
  and salt**

1 cup orange juice

1/4 cup vegetable oil

1 egg

1/4 cup raisins, *or other coarsely chopped
  dried fruit*

Preheat oven to 400°F. Lightly spray a muffin pan with nonstick cooking spray; set aside.

In a large bowl combine the bran, flours, sugar, baking powder, cinnamon, and salt; set aside. In a medium bowl or large measuring cup combine the remaining ingredients, except the raisins.

Make a well in the center of the bran mixture. Pour in the orange juice mixture. Stir until just combined; fold in the raisins. Spoon the batter evenly into the prepared muffin pan. Bake for 18 to 20 minutes, or until the muffins are golden brown. Transfer the muffins to a wire rack to cool.

NUTRITION VALUES PER MUFFIN
Calories 189.9
Fat 7.1g
Cholesterol 20.1mg
Sodium 268.9mg
Protein 3.9g
Carbohydrates 28.9g
Fiber 2.5g

Country Vegetable-Bean Soup

Serve this easy soup with a tossed salad and some crusty whole-grain bread for a very satisfying meal. That combination will also give you about a third of your fiber quota for the day.

1 15-ounce can reduced-sodium chicken broth

3 large celery ribs *(with leaves), cut in 1/2-inch slices*

2 medium carrots, *scrubbed (not peeled), and cut in 1/4-inch dice*

2 medium zucchini, *cut into 1/2-inch pieces*

2 teaspoons extra-virgin olive oil

1 1/2 teaspoons dried thyme leaves

1 16-ounce can cannellini beans, drained

1/2 teaspoon salt, *optional*

Chopped fresh basil for garnish, *optional*

In a soup pot or Dutch oven combine 2 cups of water, and all the remaining ingredients, except the beans and the salt. Cover,

Be Good to Your Gut

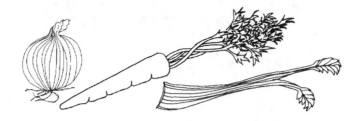

and bring to a boil. Reduce heat to low, and simmer, partially covered, for 10 minutes. Stir in the beans and the salt (if desired), and cook 10 minutes longer. Ladle into soup bowls. Garnish with basil, if desired.

TASTE TIP:

Garnish with chopped tomatoes and grated Parmesan cheese, as tolerated. Dried basil or tarragon may be used instead of the thyme.

NUTRITION VALUES PER SERVING

Calories 173.0
Fat 3.5g
Cholesterol 3.5mg
Sodium 593.4mg
Protein 8.7g
Carbohydrates 28.3g
Fiber 7.4g

Vegetarian Split Pea Soup

Makes 6 servings

You can make a savory soup using liquid natural hickory seasoning instead of the traditional ham hock. For a warm winter dinner, serve the soup with a salad and whole-grain bread. As an appetizer, it's a high-fiber way to start a meal.

1 pound split peas, *sorted and rinsed*

8 cups water *or* vegetable stock *(page 18)*

2 teaspoons natural hickory seasoning,
  optional

**2 *each* whole bay leaves and 3-inch
  cinnamon sticks**

2 medium carrots, *scrubbed and diced*

2 large celery ribs, *cut into 1/2-inch slices*

1/4 cup chopped fresh dill, *divided*

Salt and freshly ground pepper to taste, optional

In a large saucepan or Dutch oven combine the peas, water (or stock), hickory seasoning, bay leaves, and cinnamon sticks. Cover, and bring to a boil over high heat. Reduce heat, and simmer, partially covered, for 40 minutes. Add the carrots, celery and *2 tablespoons* of dill. Simmer 20 minutes longer, or until the vegetables are tender. Use a slotted spoon to remove the bay leaves and cinnamon sticks. Add the salt and pepper, if desired.

Ladle soup into bowls, and garnish with remaining dill.

TASTE TIP:

For a heartier soup, roast the vegetables (tossed with 2 teaspoons olive oil) separately in a 450°F. oven for almost 20 minutes. Cook the soup for about 50 minutes, adding the vegetables at the end.

NUTRITION VALUES PER SERVING
Calories 301.0
Fat 3.4g
Cholesterol 0.0mg
Sodium 121.6mg
Protein 19.3g
Carbohydrates 51.2g
Fiber 5.7g

Pineapple-Cucumber Salsa

Makes about 3 cups

Here's a snappy salsa to serve as an appetizer or as an enhancement to main dishes. It's a good source of fiber that can be served with vegetables, or toasted whole-wheat pita chips. It's also a nice companion to Jerk Pork Tenderloin with Black Beans (page 63).

1 20-ounce can crushed pineapple

1 small cucumber, *peeled and diced*

1 small jalapeño pepper, *seeded and diced*

3 tablespoons finely chopped cilantro

2 tablespoons rice vinegar

1 tablespoon fresh lime juice, *or to taste*

Generous pinch salt and freshly ground black pepper

In a medium bowl combine all the ingredients until blended. Cover, and let stand for about an hour to let flavors blend. Adjust seasonings if necessary.

Store in the refrigerator for later use. Bring to room temperature just before serving.

Be Good to Your Gut

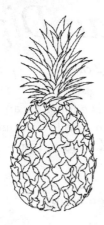

TASTE TIP:

*The jalapeño and ground black pepper
may be omitted for people with IBS or for
any others concerned with gastric irritation. Others looking for more fiber will
love this recipe.*

NUTRITION VALUES PER 1/2 CUP SERVING
Calories 77.7
Fat 0.2g
Cholesterol 0.0mg
Sodium 34.6mg
Protein 0.7g
Carbohydrates 20.8g
Fiber 1.2g

Spinach-Bean Dip

Makes 4 servings (about 2 1/2 cups)

A good tasting low-fat dip is a must for any gathering. Serve this dip in a hollowed-out red cabbage, a small round hollowed-out bread or in red bell peppers.

1 10-ounce package frozen chopped spinach

1 cup cooked garbanzo beans *or canned beans, drained*

1 cup low-fat sour cream

2 tablespoons water *or bean liquid*

1 teaspoon balsamic vinegar, *or to taste*

1/2 teaspoon *each* **onion powder and salt**

2 tablespoons chopped black olives

Cook the spinach according to package directions. Drain well, and then press out any remaining water.

In a food processor combine the spinach and beans until almost smooth; scrape down the sides of the workbowl. Add the sour cream, water (or bean liquid), vinegar, onion powder, and salt. Process just to combine or puree until smooth, if desired.

Stir in the olives. Transfer the dip to a serving bowl. Cover, and refrigerate for several hours to chill and let the flavors blend. Adjust seasonings, if desired, and serve.

TASTE TIP:

Any raw or steamed vegetable — as tolerated — goes well with this dip: celery, carrot or zucchini sticks, asparagus spears, yellow squash slices, and cherry tomatoes are colorful accompaniments.

NUTRITION VALUES PER SERVING

Calories 141.5
Fat 4.7g
Cholesterol 0.0mg
Sodium 410.5mg
Protein 5.8g
Carbohydrates 19.7g
Fiber 1.6g

Gingered Chicken

Makes 4 servings

This easy meal is loaded with fiber and color. It's also fun to make. Using broth instead of fat to stir-fry keeps both the fat and calorie count low.

1 1/2 cups reduced-sodium chicken broth, *divided*

2 teaspoons freshly grated ginger root

12 ounces skinless boneless chicken breast, *cut into 1/2-inch strips*

2 cups sliced celery

2 cups sliced mushrooms

1 cup chopped carrots

1/4 teaspoon *each* onion powder and garlic powder

1 cup snow pea pods

2 tablespoons light soy sauce

1 tablespoon dry sherry wine *or* water

1/2 teaspoon cornstarch

Hot cooked brown rice *(page 24)*

In a wok or large nonstick skillet combine 1/4 cup of the broth and the ginger. Heat until just boiling. Add the chicken, and cook, stirring constantly, for 3 minutes, or

Be Good to Your Gut

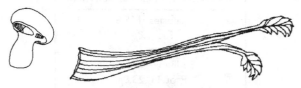

until the chicken is opaque. Remove the chicken and set aside.

Pour 1 cup of the broth into the wok or skillet. Stir in the celery, mushrooms, carrots, onion powder, and garlic powder. Stir-fry for 5 to 6 minutes. Add the pea pods, and cook for 3 to 5 minutes longer, or until the vegetables are tender-crisp.

In a small bowl stir together the remaining broth, soy sauce, sherry (or water), and cornstarch, until the cornstarch is dissolved. Pour into the vegetable mixture. Cook for 2 to 3 minutes, or until the mixture boils. Return chicken to the pan, and cook until heated through. Serve over rice.

TASTE TIP:
Other favorite and well-tolerated vegetables such as broccoli, chinese cabbage, scallions, onion, and green or red pepper can be added or substituted for the ones above.

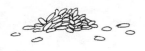

```
┌─────────────────────────────────────┐
│ NUTRITION VALUES PER SERVING          │
│ ─────────────────────────────────     │
│         Calories  165.8               │
│           Fat  1.8g                   │
│       Cholesterol  52.3mg             │
│        Sodium  445.7mg                │
│        Protein  23.8g                 │
│      Carbohydrates  12.1g             │
│         Fiber  2.7g                   │
└─────────────────────────────────────┘
```

Jerk Pork Tenderloin with Black Beans

Makes 4 servings

There's no modifying this zesty dish — the spices are what make it. Serve it with Pineapple-Cucumber Salsa (page 56). That will keep your fiber quota for the day in its upper limit. Warmed corn or flour tortillas also go well with this entree.

1 whole pork tenderloin *(about 1 1/4 pounds)*

Jerk Seasoning*

2 15-ounce cans black beans, *drained*

1 small red onion, *chopped*

2 teaspoons chili powder

1 teaspoon ground cumin

1/2 teaspoon vegetable oil

1/4 cup chopped cilantro

2 tablespoons lime juice

Salt, *to taste*

Preheat oven to 425°F.

Place the whole tenderloin in a shallow roasting pan. Sprinkle the Jerk Seasoning on all sides of the meat, turning it and pressing in the seasoning. Roast for 20 to 25 minutes, or until the internal temperature reads 155°F on a meat thermometer.

Let the pork rest for about 10 minutes to make slicing easier. (Internal temperature should rise about 5 degrees, to 160°, while resting.)

Meanwhile, in a nonstick skillet, combine the beans, onion, chili powder, cumin, oil, and 1/4 cup water. Cook over medium-high heat for about 3 minutes, or until heated through. Stir in the chopped cilantro, lime juice, and salt to taste.

Serve the sliced tenderloin with the beans.

Be Good to Your Gut

***Jerk Seasoning** Mix together 1 tablespoon dried minced onion, 2 teaspoons crushed dried thyme leaves, 1 teaspoon onion powder, 1 teaspoon *each* salt, sugar, and ground allspice, 1/4 teaspoon *each* ground nutmeg and ground cinnamon, and 1/8 teaspoon ground red pepper. (Makes enough to coat one whole pork tenderloin.)

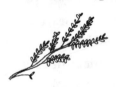

NUTRITION VALUES PER SERVING
Calories 333.9
Fat 7.7g
Cholesterol 104.0mg
Sodium 1111.2mg
Protein 44.3g
Carbohydrates 30.3g
Fiber 8.3g

Roasted Vegetables and Idaho Potatoes

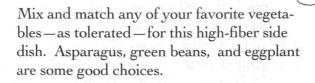

Makes 4 servings

Mix and match any of your favorite vegetables—as tolerated—for this high-fiber side dish. Asparagus, green beans, and eggplant are some good choices.

6 large mushrooms, *cleaned and quartered*

1 large Idaho potato *(unpeeled), scrubbed and cut into 1-inch cubes*

1 medium zucchini, *cut into 1-inch cubes*

1 medium yellow squash, *cut into 1-inch cubes*

1 medium red bell pepper, *seeded and cut into 1-inch cubes*

1 medium onion, *coarsely chopped*

5 teaspoons olive oil

1/2 cup crumbled Feta cheese with basil and tomato *(about 2 ounces)* *

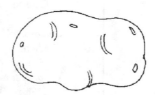

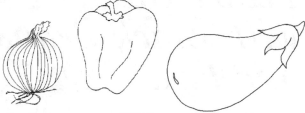

Preheat oven to 400°F.

In a large roasting pan toss together all the ingredients, except the salt, pepper, and feta. Roast for about 40 minutes, or until the vegetables are nicely browned and the potatoes are tender, stirring occasionally.

Transfer to a large platter or serving dish. Sprinkle the feta over the top. Serve hot, or at room temperature.

Feta cheese with basil and tomato is a packaged variety found in the dairy case in the supermarket.

NUTRITION VALUES PER SERVING

Calories 249.8
Fat 9.5g
Cholesterol 12.6mg
Sodium 173.7mg
Protein 8.6g
Carbohydrates 35.8g
Fiber 5.3g

Yellow Rice with Black Beans and Peas

Makes 6 servings

Use any of your favorite beans in this recipe. The black ones add a dramatic touch. This is a tasty and versatile side dish to serve with grilled chicken or meat. Vegetarians will relish this as a tasty addition to their menus as well.

2 1/4 cups reduced-sodium chicken *or* vegetable broth, divided

2 teaspoons olive oil

1 cup long-grain rice

1/2 teaspoon ground tumeric

1 15-ounce can black beans, drained

1 cup thawed, frozen baby peas

1 teaspoon ground cumin

3/4 teaspoon salt, *or* to taste

In a medium saucepan combine 2 cups of the broth, and the oil. Bring to a boil and stir in the rice and tumeric; reduce heat to low. Cover, and cook for 20 minutes, or until the rice is done and most of the water is absorbed.

Just before the rice is finished, combine the reserved broth and the remaining ingredients in a large skillet, and cook over high heat until heated through (alternately, place in a large microwavable dish and microwave on HIGH for 2 minutes).

Stir the bean mixture into the cooked rice. Serve hot, or at room temperature.

TASTE TIP:

Salsa is a tasty garnish to serve with this. You might substitute curry powder for the cumin and add a pinch of ground red pepper, as tolerated.

NUTRITION VALUES PER SERVING
Calories 127.5
Fat 3.3g
Cholesterol 3.0mg
Sodium 373.1mg
Protein 6.5g
Carbohydrates 34.2g
Fiber 3.7g

Cranberry-Yogurt Coffee Cake

Makes 14 servings

Inspired by the test kitchens of Dannon yogurt, this low-fat cake is a great snack or satisfying dessert. Cranberries and whole-wheat flour add extra fiber. Try chopped frozen cherries or your favorite dried fruit if cranberries aren't available. Some chopped nuts (if tolerated) will boost the fiber, too.

1 3/4 cups all-purpose flour

3/4 cup whole-wheat flour

2 1/2 teaspoons baking powder

3/4 teaspoon baking soda

1/4 teaspoon salt

2/3 cup honey

1/3 cup vegetable oil

1/2 cup thawed, frozen egg substitute

1 whole egg

Grated peel of 1 medium orange, *optional*

1 cup nonfat orange yogurt

1 cup coarsely chopped cranberries

Preheat oven to 350°F. Lightly spray a 9-inch bundt or ring pan with nonstick cooking spray; set aside.

In a large bowl whisk together the flours, baking powder, baking soda, and salt; set aside.

In a medium bowl, using an electric mixer on medium speed, beat the honey and oil until creamy. Add the egg substitute, egg, and orange peel (if using) and beat 1 minute longer. Add the yogurt, and beat on low speed until just blended.

Make a well in the center of the flour mixture; pour in the liquid mixture. Stir by hand just until blended. Fold in the cranberries. Pour the batter into the prepared pan; smooth the top with the back of a spoon.

Bake for 35 to 40 minutes, or until a toothpick inserted in the center of the cake comes out clean. Cool the cake in the pan on a wire rack for 10 minutes. Invert onto the rack and remove from the pan to cool completely.

NUTRITION VALUES PER SERVING

Calories 183.1
Fat 5.8g
Cholesterol 13.2mg
Sodium 192.3mg
Protein 4.3g
Carbohydrates 29.6g
Fiber 1.4g

Be Good to Your Gut

Apple-Oatmeal Crisp

Makes 8 servings

Nothing smells as good as apples baking. And this easy crisp has oatmeal, whole-wheat flour, and wheat germ for added fiber. Serve it with frozen yogurt for an extra treat.

1/2 cup rolled oats

6 tablespoons packed brown sugar, *divided*

1/4 cup whole-wheat flour

1/4 cup margarine *or* soy margarine

3 tablespoons unsweetened wheat germ

5 medium Granny Smith apples, *peeled, cored, and sliced*

1 teaspoon grated lemon peel

Preheat oven to 350°F. Lightly spray an 8-inch square baking pan with nonstick cooking spray; set aside.

In a small bowl combine the oats, 4 tablespoons of the sugar, and the flour. Cut in the margarine with a pastry cutter, or with two knives until the mixture is in coarse, pea-sized lumps; stir in the wheat germ.

Place the fruit in the baking pan and sprinkle with the remaining sugar and lemon peel. Spoon the oat mixture evenly over the top. Bake for 40 to 45 minutes, or until golden brown. Place the pan on a wire rack to cool. Serve warm.

TASTE TIP:

Use any tart, crisp apples; they will hold their shape better when cooked. One cup of pitted, chopped prunes can be added to the apples before baking for extra fiber and flavor; using unpeeled apples will add more fiber, too.

NUTRITION VALUES PER SERVING

Calories 161.7
Fat 6.7g
Cholesterol 0.0mg
Sodium 79.9mg
Protein 2.4g
Carbohydrates 25.1g
Fiber 2.9g

Be Good to Your Gut

Strawberries and Pears with Creamy Yogurt Sauce

Makes 4 servings

Use any of your favorite berries, or even kiwi fruit in this yummy dessert. Try other canned fruits to give this dessert a new look each time.

2 cups fresh strawberries, *quartered*

1 16-ounce can pear slices, *packed in juice, drained*

1 cup Creamy Yogurt Sauce, *page 26*

Fresh mint for garnish

In a medium bowl combine the strawberries and pears. Cover, and refrigerate until ready to serve. Spoon into dessert dishes, and pour an equal amount of the sauce over each. Garnish with mint leaves.

TASTE TIP:

Drizzle a little chocolate syrup or fudge sauce over the top.

NUTRITION VALUES PER SERVING

Calories 122.2
Fat 0.4g
Cholesterol 1.0mg
Sodium 46.7mg
Protein 3.1g
Carbohydrates 26.6g
Fiber 4.2g

Be Good to Your Gut

IRRITABLE BOWEL SYNDROME AND GAS

Irritable bowel syndrome (IBS) poses something of a dilemma: Physicians readily recognize when a person has it, but describing a consistent pattern of symptoms is nearly impossible. People with an irritable bowel may complain of cramping pain in any part of the abdomen, feeling bloated, "gas," constipation as well as diarrhea, and excessive mucus in the stool—singly or in any combination! Often, the same person may complain of either constipation or diarrhea, later experience the other symptom, and then alternate again. The symptom that occurs most frequently also will vary from individual to individual.

Worldwide, IBS affects about 1 in 7 to 1 in 10 people. Over 22 million Americans suffer from this condition, which is second only to the common cold as a cause of absenteeism from work. Reports indicate that three times as many women as men are afflicted with irritable bowel syndrome. Researchers speculate that the fluctuation of reproductive hormones during menstrual cycles may increase the occurrence of these symptoms. The truth is that the cause or causes of IBS are not well understood at all. It is very likely that multiple factors are involved.

You can guess at the number of disorders that researchers thought produced IBS by ticking off the names given to this problem over the years. Irritable bowel syndrome has been called psychogenic *colitis*, mucous *colitis*, or just plain *colitis* — suggesting that there is inflammation (or "-itis") of the lining of the colon. This is a misnomer because no inflammation is present.

Perhaps, as some have suggested, if there is an inflammation it is is due to a bowel infection. Nowadays, most physicians do not believe infection is a factor. They do think, though, that some irritation of the small or large intestine is involved.

Irritable bowel syndrome has also been called *psychogenic* colitis, or the *nervous* gut, in the belief that psychologic distress — "nerves," depression, or anxiety — causes the onset of symptoms.

At one time, intolerance to certain foods and food allergies were considered major factors in IBS. While we do not know that this is not the case, it is unlikely to be the only cause.

Another name for IBS was *spastic* colitis or *spastic* colon. This referred to the painful contractions a sufferer would feel inside his or her lower gut. These abnormal, uncoordinated contractions, or dysmotility, may be linked to a change in the "firing" of electrical signals that control muscular activity. This "pacemaker" mechanism is similar to the system controlling the contraction of heart muscle. And as with the heart, an abnormal pattern or rhythm — a *dysrhythmia* — may develop.

Recent research has strongly suggested a central role for abnormal gut sensitivity. According to this view, motility in the gut is normal. However, the nerve endings in the lining of the small and large intestines are unusually sensitive and will react abnormally to even ordinary events such as eating. For example, when ingested food reaches the bowel, the gut wall expands (or distends), causing the nerves to trigger exaggerated patterns of muscular activity. As a result, sometimes, a meal may be followed almost immediately by cramps, and soon after by a bowel movement. Other stimuli that can cause this over-reacting include stressful events, taking certain medications, drinking milk or swallowing too much air.

In any person with irritable bowel syndrome, it is difficult to pin down the cause because each time, the underlying disorder, or combination of contributing disorders, will probably be different. Thus, there is no specific test you can take that will tell whether or not you have IBS — and no procedure that will allow the physician to see what is wrong. In technical language, that means IBS is a *functional* disorder.

Nevertheless, your physician will frequently order tests, because your symptoms might suggest the presence of another, more serious disease. He or she will be particularly alert to this possibility if you have rectal bleeding, weight loss, or severe, persistent pain. After analyzing the results of appropriate tests, the physician will be able to reassure you, for example, that you do not have cancer.

What to Do about It

Even though we do not fully understand the causes of irritable bowel syndrome, dietary recommendations and techniques for reducing stress, along with the use of medications for specific symptoms, have been shown to work for a substantial number of people. Both diet and stress can be managed quite well. For example, adding more fiber, drinking lots of water, and a following a moderate exercise program may do the trick for some. Others may need to keep a food diary for a few days to target problem foods, or learn to deal with stress situations through counseling.

Diet Fat seems to be a major offender in exacerbating IBS, because in any form it is a strong stimulus of colonic contractions. So, foods such as cream, cheese, vegetable oils, shortening of any kind, avocados, whipped toppings, and meat will need a reevaluation. It's not necessary to eliminate any of them altogether. However, it is helpful to know exactly how much of each item you're eating. With that information in hand, you can begin to make some small modifications. Start by reducing portion sizes, using less rich sauces with main dishes, and having more high-fiber foods at meals and as snacks.

Chocolate, caffeine, alcohol, and milk products are also frequent offenders. Yogurt and other cultured products may not give any distress at all.

For a while, you'll have to keep a journal noting the foods that seem to cause the most problems. The latest research indicates that fructose (a sugar found in fruit) and sorbitol (an artificial sweetener) may aggravate IBS symptoms. That may be why apple, grape, and pear juices are linked with diarrhea and abdominal pain. Excessive intake of magnesium-containing antacids also can cause diarrhea.

In many people with IBS who predominantly have constipation, dietary fiber seems to offer relief (see page 33). Increase your fiber intake gradually, and eat just enough so that you have a soft and easily passed bowel movement. Fruits, vegetables, whole-grain cereals and breads, lentils, and beans all are good sources of dietary fiber. Six to 11 servings of breads, cereals, and grains; 3 to 5 servings of vegetables; and 2 to 4 servings of fruits are the recommendations in the *Dietary Guidelines for Americans* and the *Food Guide Pyramid*. In addition, you might want to include about three tablespoons of bran each day with meals. Start with one tablespoon of bran once or twice a day, and work your way up from there.

Reduce or eliminate any foods that you already know cause distress for you. Beans, for instance, are usually not well tolerated by people with IBS. Other gas-producing foods, such as cabbage or grapes, also may be a problem.

Strange as it may seem, high-fiber diets can also help when diarrhea is the major symptom. The basic water-holding ability of fiber helps to absorb excess fluids and also to increase the bulk of the stool. Those two actions are beneficial in regulating colonic motility. That regulation, or adjustment, means a stabilizing effect for both constipation and diarrhea.

On the other hand, there *are* a few individuals in whom fiber may intensify constipation or diarrhea. For them, high-fiber foods should be eliminated from the diet. It's a good idea to talk to your doctor or dietitian first. Even if you're not one of these individuals, it's possible you may have added too much fiber too soon; your system may not have yet had the opportunity to adjust to the presence of extra fiber.

Cramping and diarrhea can be brought on by large meals. So, try to eat smaller meals throughout the day, or reduce the total amount you eat. In addition, select foods that are low in fat and high in fiber. While you're at it, learn to chew your food thoroughly, and allow enough time to eat your meals slowly and in a relaxed way.

Make sure to drink plenty of water as you begin to increase your fiber intake. Six to 8 glasses of water a day — probably more than you're drinking now — should be the goal. The extra fluid will also keep you well hydrated and feeling better throughout the day. You'll want to avoid carbonated water (or other drinks), especially with meals. These can produce "gas" and lead to discomfort.

In fact, you may even want to avoid sipping plain water during meals because which facilitate the swallowing of air and also increase gas. Make a habit of drinking water in the early and mid mornings and afternoons.

You may want to identify foods that you suspect you're allergic to or don't tolerate well. In some people, citrus fruits, gluten, eggs, or chocolate may produce reactions. Note, though, that lactose is less often an offender than is commonly believed. And a person with true intolerance can readily find low-lactose dairy products, as well as lactase supplements which will facilitate the digestion of lactose in food. Have a look at page 221 if you believe you are lactose intolerant. The information there will help you to evaluate what really may be going on, as well as offer you suggestions for including dairy foods in your diet again.

Stress Stress—whether it be related to business, career, marriage, family, fear of a dreaded disease, or sexual difficulties—seems to increase colonic spasms, especially in people with IBS. A true cause-and-effect relationship has yet to be demonstrated, but the evidence in support of a connection is strong. Certainly, irritable bowel symptoms increase during periods of anxiety, depression, or panic. Fortunately, stress-reducing techniques are available. The bonus is that these methods also can help enhance your daily life.

Biofeedback, hypnosis, meditation, and psychological counseling are the most common stress-reducing techniques to help you cope with IBS. The first is a system that

trains patients to monitor—and improve—
their health by learning to recognize signals
from their own bodies. It is also quite helpful in teaching people how to relax.
Initially, biofeedback involves the use of
equipment that picks up electrical signals in
the muscles. It also requires the services of
a certified biofeedback therapist, who may
also be a physician or a psychotherapist.
(See Resources, page 231, for more information.)

Hypnosis is a centuries-old practice that
is receiving new attention. The American
Medical Association has approved hypnosis
training since 1958, and today many health
care professionals use this approach to help
people with weight problems, cigarette
smoking, and chronic stress. Because hypnosis is a state of heightened suggestibility
brought on by increased relaxation, people
can learn a variety of ways to deal with
stress-related behavioral patterns.

Hypnosis seems to hold great potential
for those suffering from IBS. One study
showed a clinical improvement in 85% of
patients under 50 years of age. Be sure
you're working with a well-trained,
licensed hypnotherapist. Again, he or she
may be a physician, a psychologist, or a
nurse-practitioner. Try to obtain a personal
referral or contact the American Institute
of Hypnotherapy (See Resources, page
231). Most important of all, have a positive

attitude. Self-motivation is helpful in changing any behavior.

Other Suggestions Daily exercise is a great way to reduce stress, and it makes people feel better psychologically as well as physically. Allow enough time for regular bowel movements. Trying to postpone a movement or rushing it will only cause more anxiety. That, in turn, will aggravate your symptoms. Relaxation, as mentioned before, is an important key to the successful management of irritable bowel syndrome.

Sometimes drugs can help provide symptomatic relief. However, know that no one medication will be effective in everyone with IBS. If an individual mostly has diarrhea, his or her physician may recommend loperamide (Imodium®), or, on rare occasions cholestyramine (Questran®). If severe constipation is the primary problem, consider taking natural vegetable fiber like bran or psyllium. Try food sources of fiber before buying an over-the-counter fiber supplement. In some individuals with constipation, a promotility drug—that is, one of a class of drugs that strengthen muscular contractions, such as cisapride (Propulsid®)—can be useful by increasing the number of bowel movements and reducing laxative use.

To treat debilitating pain, the physician may consider a tricyclic antidepressant. For chronic abdominal pain that presents after

meals, part of the treatment may be administration beforehand of an anticholinergic
agent—a drug that inhibits the nerves regulating intestinal contractions.

Finally, bear in mind that treatments for
irritable bowel syndrome are personal and
depend entirely on the individual. Spend
some time identifying what is irritating your
individual system. Then develop an approach
that can effect lifestyle changes — diet, exercise, and stress reduction — on a gradual
basis. Modifications that can be adopted step
by step in a comfortable manner are the ones
that are most effective and long-lasting.

Reducing Fat

It is helpful to know a few quick tricks
that can help keep fat out of your meal
while maintaining good flavor.

- Choose low-fat cuts of meat and chicken
  in the supermarket.

- Try to roast, broil, poach, stir-fry, or
  microwave when cooking at home. Look
  for some terms like "roasted" or "broiled"
  in restaurants instead of ordering foods
  that are sautéed or fried.

- Use broths, juices, water, and/or wine to
  steam vegetables, poultry, and fish instead
  of sautéing in oil.

- In restaurants, ask the server whether the fish or meat is marinated in oil before it is grilled. If it is, request that it be cooked with little or no oil.

- Select low- and nonfat dairy products. Use the higher fat cheeses like gorgonzola, or an aged cheddar in small quantities to perk up the flavor in a grain or pasta dish.

- Invest in a new microwave oven, high quality pressure cooker, or nonstick wok. All of these devices cook food fast and with little fat and oil.

- Cook quantities of rice, beans, and grains; then freeze in small portions (use zip-lock bags or plastic bowls). These foods defrost quickly or they can be tossed (while still frozen) into soups and sauces.

- Puree leftover beans or vegetables with a bit of salt and your favorite herb (basil, perhaps) to use as a tasty replacement for butter or cream cheese.

- Read labels. The new food label format makes it easier than ever to know exactly how much fat is in one portion of that food. Consider how may portions you'll really be eating. However, don't automatically pass up an item if it appears to have a large percentage of fat calories. Consider what else you're eating throughout the day. Balance is the key.

How Much Fat?

The recommendations of the *U.S. Dietary Guidelines for Americans* and a number of other health organizations are quite consistent. Fat should represent 30 percent, or less, of your total daily calories. For most people that concept doesn't mean too much. However, if you consider that most adults consume between 1,500 and 2,400 calories a day, the range for fat should be 50 to 80 grams for the day. Once you choose your number of total fat grams, then try to keep the amount of *saturated* fat—the kind that comes from animal products—to a third or less of the total amount. For example, if 60 grams is your total fat allowance, keep saturated fat to 20 grams or less per day.

You can be the judge of how many total grams to have each day. Part of that may depend on how severe your IBS is, and what your weight goals are. A registered dietitian can help you plan a menu that is best suited to your lifestyle and personal needs. There is also some flexibility here. Most dietitians today will have you look at a weekly pattern, rather than one day or one meal. In other words, unless you are suffering intense distress, a little more fat on one day can be balanced out with less the next. This is another situation in which a food diary can come in handy. Keeping a record of several days of normal eating will give a clearer picture of how much fat you're currently eating. That makes it easier to make any adjustments if they're necessary.

Food labels are quite clear about the number of grams contained in one serving. Just be sure to calculate properly if you're actually eating several servings. There are also a number of nifty little fat-counter books around. They list a wide variety of all the food categories with the amounts of fat in specific items; frequently they include calorie and cholesterol information as well. They're a good way to start getting acquainted with the amount of fat that's in your favorite foods.

Intestinal Gas and Flatulence

People with irritable bowel syndrome are particularly bothered by the pain, discomfort, and embarrassment of "gas." Whether that gas is coming from above the belt or below, it's still a nuisance. Knowing more about gas can help make its management easier. In most cases, it should be possible to reduce its occurrence considerably.

Basically there are three sources of intestinal gas. Every day each one of us produces about 10 liters (or some 10 quarts) of gas. Normally, most of the gas is absorbed through the bowel wall into the bloodstream. People with irritable bowel syndrome don't produce more gas than others. The discomfort may make it feel that way, but actually the amount of gas produced in people doesn't vary considerably. It probably feels more painful to someone with IBS because that person is more sensitive to normal degrees of abdominal distention and because there may be abnormal intestinal motility.

Room air is another source of gas. Most of the time, too much air is swallowed ("aerophagia") while eating or drinking. Aerophagia may be a nervous habit, related to anxiety. Gulping food, chewing gum, chewing with your mouth open, and drinking carbonated beverages are other means by which too much air gets into the stomach. The result is belching, the most common symptom of gas. Excess air can cause further discomfort if you wear tight clothes or lie down soon after a meal. If the air isn't released through belching, then bloating and abdominal discomfort result.

Gas expelled through the rectum (flatulence) is usually caused by fermentation of food by "friendly" bacteria normally present in the intestine. These bacteria frequently act on indigestible carbohydrates like those found in beans, dried peas, and lentils. Fruits and grains, which are also high in fiber, can have the same effect. Other food sources that may cause flatulence include milk and other dairy products (see page 221); fructose, a fruit sugar which is used as a sweetener in foods and beverages and which may be incompletely digested; and sorbitol and mannitol, two artificial sweeteners. Flatulence also can be caused by certain medicines like colestipol (Colestid®), which is used to lower blood cholesterol levels.

What to Do about It

Diet Avoid gas-producing foods like those listed on page 94. Once again, the food diary becomes a handy tool for identifying offending foods. Remember that what bothers one person may not bother another. The quantity of food or beverage ingested may be a factor. For instance, someone may experience pain after eating two cups of beans, yet be fine with a half-cup serving.

For nutrition's sake, don't just randomly eliminate foods from your diet. Take some care to find alternative solutions as well. For instance, if beans are irritating, consider using Beano®, a nonprescription product containing alpha-galactosidase, an enzyme which breaks down the carbohydrates in beans that most people find bothersome. Note: this is added to foods *as well as* swallowed or chewed. Another possible solution for reducing intestinal gas is to soak the beans overnight and discard the soaking water before cooking. Adding fiber slowly to the diet and drinking plenty of water along the way are the best means of avoiding excess flatulence. Though not systematically studied, regular exercise has been reported to aid in relieving or preventing gas.

Other Suggestions Relaxation techniques may be helpful in reducing the amount of air swallowed if the problem is related to stress. Other remedies include eating fewer hard candies, reducing the amount of carbonated beverages you drink, and even talking less when you eat. Finally, over-the-counter products like simethicone (Mylicon®) and simethicone-containing antacid preparations may be effective in breaking-up trapped gas.

Possible Gas Producing Foods:

The real list of problem foods is potentially endless because everyone's body responds to food differently. Here's a list of the foods that most commonly cause distress.

Fruits:

Apples (raw)
Apple juice
Avocado
Bananas
Cantaloupe
Honeydew
Grapes
Raisins
Watermelon

Misc.:

Carbonated
  beverages
Chewing gum
Hard candy
Nuts
Mannitol and
  Sorbitol —
  synthetic
  sweeteners
Fats and high fat
  foods
Rich sauces,
  gravies

Vegetables:

Beans (kidney, lima, navy)
Broccoli
Brussels sprouts
Cabbage
Cauliflower
Corn
Cucumbers
Leeks

Onions
Split peas
Lentils
Peppers, green
Radishes
Scallions
Shallots
Soybeans

Cereals and Grains:

Bran Cereals
Excessive quantities of wheat products

RECIPES

Banana-Nut Muffins

Seviche

Steve's Meatloaf

Baked Stuffed Salmon

Smoked Chicken and
Brown Rice Salad

Whole-Wheat Angel Hair Pasta
with Fresh Vegetables

Barley-Fennel Pilaf

Apple-Nut Stuffed Squash

Rice Confetti

Sherried Fruit Compote

Pretty Pink Applesauce

Banana-Nut Muffins

Makes 6 muffins

These muffins smell great and taste delicious plain or with diet margarine or sugar-free fruit spreads. They make a nutritious start to the day.

1 cup mashed bananas (about 2 medium)

1/2 cup thawed frozen apple juice concentrate

2 tablespoons canola oil

1 1/4 cups rice flour

1 1/2 teaspoons baking powder

1/4 cup pignoli nuts

Preheat oven to 375°F. Lightly spray a muffin pan with nonstick cooking spray; set aside.

In a medium bowl, combine the banana, apple juice concentrate, and oil. In a separate bowl, whisk together the flour and baking powder.

Be Good to Your Gut

Make a well in the center of the flour
mixture. Pour in the apple juice mixture.
Stir until just combined, then fold in the
nuts. Spoon the batter evenly into the
prepared muffin pan. Bake for 20 to 25
minutes, or until the muffins are golden
brown. Transfer the muffins to a wire rack
to cool.

TASTE TIP:
*For a fun and flavorful change, substitute
tangerine juice and chopped pecans. For
extra fiber, add 1/4 cup raisins or dates.*

NUTRITION VALUES PER MUFFIN

Calories 278.9
Fat 10.2g
Cholesterol 0.0mg
Sodium 119.2g
Protein 3.4g
Carbohydrates 46.5g
Fiber 2.2g

Seviche

Makes 4 servings

Spanish people have known for centuries that most fish can be "cooked" just by marinating it in lemon juice until it is opaque and slightly firm. Here is an easy way to sample it in your own kitchen.

1/2 pound sea scallops

1/3 cup fresh lemon juice

1/2 cup chopped celery

2 tablespoons sliced green olives

1 tablespoon chopped fresh chives

2 teaspoons olive oil

1/2 teaspoon *each* dried oregano leaves and onion powder

1/4 teaspoon salt

4 cups chopped lettuce

Wash and dry the scallops; cut each one in half.

In a medium glass bowl combine the scallops and lemon juice (add additional juice if it does not cover the scallops). Cover, and refrigerate for about 3 hours, or until the scallops are white and opaque, indicating that they are "cooked."

Add the remaining ingredients and toss gently until combined. Cover, and refrigerate until ready to serve. Place lettuce leaves on 4 serving plates; top each with an equal amount of seviche, and serve.

TASTE TIP:

Add 1/2 cup each tomatoes and onions, if tolerated. The addition of warm crusty French bread is essential for getting every last bit of the flavorful juices.

NUTRITION VALUES PER SERVING
Calories 104.6
Fat 3.7g
Cholesterol 30.1mg
Sodium 403.1mg
Protein 14.0g
Carbohydrates 5.7g
Fiber 0.9g

Steve's Meat Loaf

Makes 8 servings

Adding mixed vegetables to the ground meat adds fiber to this tasty meat loaf. The combination of ground turkey and extra-lean beef keeps the fat and cholesterol at a sane level. As simple as this recipe is, it is quite delicious. Leftovers make great sandwiches. Serve it with some nonfat gravy or salsa (if tolerated).

1 pound ground turkey

1 pound ground extra-lean beef

1 16-ounce can mixed vegetables, *drained*

3/4 cup seasoned bread crumbs

1/2 cup thawed frozen egg substitute

Preheat oven to 350°F.

In a medium bowl, combine all the ingredients until blended; don't overmix or meat loaf will be dry. Gently pack the meat into an 8 x 4 x 2 1/2-inch loaf pan. Bake for about 1 hour, or until a meat thermometer inserted in the center of the loaf reads 160°F.

Pour off any accumulated fat. Let the loaf stand for 10 minutes before slicing.

NUTRITION VALUES PER SERVING

Calories 283.8
Fat 9.0g
Cholesterol 77.9mg
Sodium 519.2mg
Protein 33.2g
Carbohydrates 16.5g
Fiber 2.2g

Baked Stuffed Salmon

Makes 8 servings

This is an easy and delicious way to increase your fiber intake. Outdoor grill enthusiasts can cook the salmon over hot coals for about 15 to 17 minutes per side. Use a fish-grilling basket to turn fish or wrap it securely in aluminum foil.

1 **whole salmon,** *butterflied* * *(about 4 pounds)*

1 **lemon,** *thinly sliced, and pitted*

1 **small zucchini,** *thinly sliced*

1 **small yellow squash,** *thinly sliced*

1 **medium onion,** *cut into thin rings* *

2 **tablespoons chopped fresh parsley**

1 **teaspoon dried dill weed**

1/2 **teaspoon salt**

2 **tablespoons margarine *or* soy margarine**

1 **teaspoon canola oil**

Parsley sprigs and additional lemon slices for garnish

Preheat oven to 400°F.

Be Good to Your Gut

Open the fish out in a large shallow baking dish. Place alternating layers of lemon and vegetables on one side of the fish, starting with the lemon.

Sprinkle with herbs and salt and dot with small pieces of margarine. Close the fish and secure it with toothpicks. Rub the fish lightly with oil. Bake for about 25 to 30 minutes, or until the fish flakes easily when tested with a fork. Garnish with lemon slices and sprigs of parsley, if desired.

* To butterfly a fish, remove the backbone with a sharp knife without splitting the fish in half. Remember to remove the row of pin bones along the sides of the fish.

TASTE TIP:
Omit the onion if necessary and sprinkle the layers of vegetables with 1/2 to 1 teaspoon of onion powder. Good substitutes for salmon are striped bass, red snapper, fresh water bass, or your favorite whole fish.

NUTRITION VALUES PER SERVING

Calories 362.4
Fat 17.7g
Cholesterol 123.2mg
Sodium 267.3mg
Protein 45.2g
Carbohydrates 4.0g
Fiber 0.6g

Be Good to Your Gut

Smoked Chicken and Brown Rice Salad

Makes 4 servings

Keep bags of cooked brown rice in the freezer. They thaw in just minutes and are ready to be made into this snazzy salad. If you make this salad in advance, store the dressing in a separate container in the refrigerator. Then toss it with the other ingredients just before serving.

1/2 cup nonfat mayonnaise

1/2 cup nonfat plain yogurt

3 tablespoons cider vinegar

1 1/4 teaspoons dried tarragon leaves

1/4 teaspoon salt

4 cups cooked brown rice

1 cup sliced celery

2 medium kiwis, *peeled and coarsely chopped*

8 ounces smoked chicken, *cut into 2-inch julienne strips*

Green leaf lettuce leaves

In a small bowl whisk together the mayonnaise, yogurt, vinegar, tarragon, and salt; set aside.

In a large bowl combine the rice, celery, kiwi, and chicken. Pour the reserved dressing over the top; toss well to combine.

Arrange the lettuce leaves on a large serving platter. Mound the salad on top.

TASTE TIP:

Add any of your favorite vegetables to increase the fiber. Carrots, zucchini, and asparagus are good choices. Chopped red onion tastes nice in this salad, if tolerated.

NUTRITION VALUES PER SERVING

Calories 372.8
Fat 3.6g
Cholesterol 51.7mg
Sodium 233.3mg
Protein 20.2g
Carbohydrates 54.6g
Fiber 5.1g

Be Good to Your Gut

Whole-Wheat Angel Hair Pasta with Fresh Vegetables

Makes 4 servings

Whole-wheat pasta, in addition to its higher fiber, also has a delicious, nutty flavor. If you've never tried Portobello mushrooms you're in for a delightful surprise — their full and "meaty" texture. Longer cooking time brings out the flavor of these mushrooms.

8 ounces whole-wheat angel hair pasta

1 small zucchini, *cut in 1-inch cubes*

1 small yellow squash, *cut in 1-inch cubes*

4 tablespoons olive oil

2 large Portobello mushrooms, *coarsely chopped*

2 tablespoons chopped fresh basil

1/2 teaspoon *each* garlic salt and onion salt

Freshly grated Parmesan cheese, *as desired*

In a large pot of boiling water cook the pasta, zucchini, and squash for 6 to 8 minutes, or until pasta is al dente. Do not overcook.

Meanwhile, in a large nonstick skillet heat 1 tablespoon of the oil over medium-high heat. Cook the mushrooms for 8 to 10 minutes, or until wilted. Stir in the basil, the garlic salt, and the onion salt.

Drain the pasta and vegetables, reserving some of the cooking liquid. Add the remaining oil and the pasta-vegetable mixture to the mushrooms. Toss lightly to combine (add a little of the reserved cooking liquid if it appears too dry). Sprinkle with cheese if desired.

TASTE TIP:

Regular fresh mushrooms can be substituted for the Portobello mushrooms. You'll need about 8 ounces sliced.

NUTRITION VALUES PER SERVING
Calories 334.0
Fat 14.5g
Cholesterol 0.0mg
Sodium 459.0mg
Protein 9.5gg
Carbohydrates 46.1g
Fiber 7.6g

Be Good to Your Gut

Barley-Fennel Pilaf

Makes 6 servings

Barley is an excellent source of fiber, B vitamins, and vitamin E. Fennel gives the pilaf a sophisticated blend of flavor and texture.

1 small fennel bulb, *washed and trimmed*

1 tablespoon canola oil

1 cup uncooked barley

4 cups reduced-sodium chicken broth

1/2 teaspoon salt

1 teaspoon grated lemon peel

2 tablespoons chopped fresh parsley

Cut the fennel bulb into quarters; remove the core. Cut each quarter into very thin slices.

In a large nonstick skillet heat the oil over medium-high heat. Cook fennel for 4 to 5 minutes. Stir in the barley, broth, and salt. Bring to a boil. Cover, and reduce heat to low. Simmer for 40 to 45 minutes, or until the barley is cooked and most of the liquid is absorbed, stirring occasionally. Sprinkle with the lemon peel and parsley, and serve.

NUTRITION VALUES PER SERVING

Calories 156.2
Fat 3.2g
Cholesterol 5.3mg
Sodium 243.7mg
Protein 5.1g
Carbohydrates 27.6g
Fiber 5.3g

Be Good to Your Gut

Apple-Nut Stuffed Squash

Makes 4 servings

This is a great way to give a lift to your complex carbohydrate and fiber quota. This dish is a smashing accompaniment to chicken or turkey—especially when the meat is cooked on an outdoor grill.

2 medium acorn squash

1 apple (unpeeled), *cored and chopped*

2 teaspoons canola oil

2 cups cooked brown rice

1/4 cup chopped walnuts

1/4 cup chopped dates

1 tablespoon light maple syrup

Preheat oven to 350°. Lightly spray a baking sheet with nonstick cooking spray; set aside.

Wash squash. Cut in half and remove seeds. Place squash cut side down on the prepared baking sheet. Bake for about 30 minutes, or until tender.

In a medium nonstick skillet heat the oil over medium-high heat. Cook the apple for 3 to 4 minutes, or until almost tender. Stir in the remaining ingredients.

When the squash is cooked, turn it cut side up and fill it with the rice mixture. Cover with aluminum foil, and bake for 10 minutes longer, or until heated through.

TASTE TIP:

Substitute honey for the maple syrup and almonds or pecans for the walnuts.

NUTRITION VALUES PER SERVING

Calories 313.5
Fat 8.2g
Cholesterol 0.0mg
Sodium 23.6mg
Protein 5.6g
Carbohydrates 59.8g
Fiber 8.8g

Be Good to Your Gut

Rice Confetti

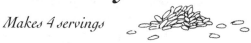

Makes 4 servings

The colorful bits of fruit add color, flavor, and texture—as well as fiber—to everyday rice. This dish is nice served with grilled meat and fish and also makes a flavorful stuffing for roast chicken.

2 1/2 cups water

1 cup long-grain rice

1 cup dried mixed fruit bits

1 teaspoon margarine *or* soy margarine

1/8 teaspoon ground cloves, optional

In a medium saucepan bring the water to a boil. Stir in the rice, fruit, margarine, and cloves (if using). Cover, and reduce heat to low. Cook for 20 minutes, or until the rice is done and most of the water is absorbed.

TASTE TIP:

You can also prepare this with brown rice. Increase water to 2 3/4 cups and cooking time to 45 to 50 minutes.

NUTRITION VALUES PER SERVING
Calories 173.8
Fat 2.4g
Cholesterol 0.0mg
Sodium 44.3mg
Protein 4.3g
Carbohydrates 59.6g
Fiber 4.6g

Be Good to Your Gut

Sherried Fruit Compote

Makes 6 servings

This simple dessert is not only easy to prepare, but it can also be made the day before.
That's especially helpful for busy schedules
or for entertaining. Dried fruit is an excellent source of fiber and a way to get extra
vitamin A and iron, too. Try serving this,
sprinkled with the orange rind, in stemmed
dessert glasses.

2 cups water

1/2 cup sherry wine

1/2 cup packed dark brown sugar

1 11 1/2-ounce package mixed dried fruit*

Grated orange rind, *optional*

6 slices fat-free golden loaf cake

In a medium saucepan combine the water,
wine, and sugar and bring to a boil. Stir in
the fruit (and orange rind, if using). Reduce
heat to low, and cook for 15 to 20 minutes,
or until the fruit is tender. Remove from
heat. Serve warm with loaf cake.

If the compote is made in advance, transfer to a glass bowl or jar. Cover, and refrigerate until ready to use.

*Note that prunes in dried fruit mixtures have pits! Remove before cooking or caution guests.

TASTE TIP:

Port wine can be substituted for the sherry for a change of pace. To eliminate wine, substitute water or your favorite fruit juice. Lemon rind may be used in place of the orange rind.

NUTRITION VALUES PER SERVING

Calories 327.9
Fat 0.0g
Cholesterol 0.0mg
Sodium 99.8mg
Protein 3.0g
Carbohydrates 75.8g
Fiber 5.2g

Be Good to Your Gut

Pretty Pink Applesauce

Makes 4 servings

Leaving the skin on apples gives a rosy hue to homemade applesauce. Fresh plums make the loveliest and freshest tasting applesauce ever, while pears add texture and body. All, you'll note, with no added sugar.

1 1/2 pounds Cortland, Winesap *or* Jonathan apples, *cored and quartered (about 4 medium)*

1 pound Santa Rosa plums, *pitted and quartered (about 4 medium)*

1 pound pears, peeled, *cored, and quartered (about 2 medium)*

1 cup water

2 tablespoons fresh lemon juice

1 cinnamon stick, *3-inches long*

In a large saucepan combine all the ingredients. Bring to a boil over high heat. Reduce heat, and partially cover. Simmer, stirring occasionally, for about 30 minutes, or until the fruit has softened. Remove the cinnamon stick. (Gently break up the fruit with the back of a spoon as it begins to soften while cooking.) Put the fruit, with its juices, through a food mill or press through a sieve.

NUTRITION VALUES PER SERVING
Calories 232.8
Fat 1.8g
Cholesterol 0.0mg
Sodium 1.9mg
Protein 1.7g
Carbohydrates 58.9g
Fiber 9.1g

Be Good to Your Gut

HEARTBURN

Heartburn. It's the bane of many Americans' existence. Heartburn and associated symptoms afflict more than 50% of all adults in this country at least once a month. And according to a 1995 Gallup survey of 1,500 respondents, 14% of all symptomatic adults have heartburn *every* day.

Heartburn, the burning sensation behind the breastbone that can flare up after a meal, is due to a backwash (known as reflux) of the stomach's contents. Ingested food triggers the stomach to produce hydrochloric acid, which helps to break down certain foods. The mixture of food and acid, along with a digestive enzyme called pepsin, refluxes up into the lower esophagus. Irritation and, in some patients, inflammation of the lining can result from extended exposure to the acid and pepsin.

Heartburn is a specific symptom of a disorder called gastroesophageal reflux disease, or GERD. That means, your heartburn is the result of the mixture of food plus acid (called chyme) backing up (*refluxing*) from the stomach (*gastro-*) into the *esophagus*.

I've already mentioned that refluxed stomach acid causes people discomfort. Did you know that reflux happens in healthy people? The difference, though, is that most of the time several muscular contractions—or motility factors—are at work to keep the esophageal lining out of harm's way. It's when these factors are not working properly in people with heartburn that GERD is considered a *motility disorder*.

The most important barrier guarding against the stomach's contents refluxing up is the tight ring of muscle at the far end of the esophagus. This lower esophageal sphincter (LES), to give the scientific name, relaxes to allow ingested food to be propelled into the stomach after swallowing. It appears that the LES also relaxes to enable upward movement of the stomach chyme, but in general it is the primary barrier against reflux. In people with GERD the LES may be weakened.

Once the stomach content comes into contact with the esophageal lining, another protective mechanism comes into play: clearance by the esophagus. This consists mainly of muscular contractions, called *peristalsis*, that push contents back into the stomach, aided by swallowed saliva which contains bicarbonate to neutralize the stomach acid. In people with heartburn, the force or frequency of contractions of the esophagus may be diminished.

If stomach muscles are working properly, ingested food is churned, partially digested by enzymes, and then transported, also by peristalsis, out of the stomach. However, the rate of stomach emptying may be decreased for a number of reasons. Slowed stomach emptying results in a greater volume of stomach content that can be refluxed, as well as greater stomach distention, which can exert pressure against the LES to make it open.

The increase in abdominal pressure that can weaken the LES may also explain the 25% frequency of *daily* heartburn in pregnant women, especially during the later part of pregnancy. The defective LES is due to increased pressure exerted by the enlarged uterus.

Thus far, three motility factors have been identified as primary causes of reflux disease. These factors may be influenced by the foods we eat. In addition to the role played by stomach acid and pepsin, there is evidence to suggest that a slippage of part of the esophagus upward into the chest through a "hole" in the diaphragm, known as a hiatus hernia, also contributes to the development of reflux symptoms. And just as GERD has multiple causes, it also has multiple symptoms: the most characteristic symptom is heartburn.

Other common complaints include regurgitation, or the rise of stomach contents into the mouth; belching; and difficulty in swallowing. Nighttime heartburn can be particularly bothersome, awakening people from sleep. In fact, according to the 1995 Gallup survey, 62% of people with heartburn say they experience their reflux symptoms at night. When stomach emptying is slow, the heartburn sufferer may also complain of an early sensation of fullness after eating only a few bites, a bloating feeling after meals, nausea, and other symptoms.

Signs of serious GERD include inflammation of the esophageal lining (esophagitis), permanent narrowing of the lumen (stricture), and bleeding. Other symptoms, like chest pain and wheezing, originate in the chest and can resemble heart or pulmonary diseases.

If, after taking a history and physical examination, the physician suspects the presence of GERD, the patient may be evaluated further, sometimes with the use of x-rays (called an upper GI series) or an endoscopy. Endoscopy is a procedure in which a small lit tube with a tiny video camera on the end (endoscope) is placed into the esophagus, enabling the doctor to view the lining for injury. Note that a substantial number of people with heartburn have no esophagitis.

What to Do about It

For the great majority of heartburn sufferers, the key to successful symptom control is adherence to some important lifestyle
changes. These include dietary recommendations, weight control, avoiding certain
medications, and sleeping with the head ele-
vated. These measures may be supplement-
ed by occasional antacid use and administration of prescription medications.

Diet Fat both weakens the LES and slows stomach emptying. Because of this double
effect, eating too much fat is a major factor
in the development of heartburn. Thus,
simply limiting the number of times you
have fat-rich meats, sauces, gravies, dressings, pastries, and cheeses will go a long
way toward relieving your distress. Try to
reduce the amounts of butter, mayonnaise,
and whole-milk dairy products you have at
each meal or as part of your snacks.
Needless to say, the less fried food you eat,
the better you're likely to feel.

Try to include lean meats, poultry, fish,
skim or low-fat milk, yogurt, and low-fat ice
cream in your diet. Carbohydrate foods like
rice, pasta, and potatoes are other good
choices. The important part is to prepare
these foods with little or no added fat.

Other foods that affect the LES the wrong way and exacerbate heartburn are chocolate, alcohol, peppermint, and spearmint. You should reduce your consumption of these items, as well as of coffee, citrus juices, tomatoes, and tomato-based foods and sauces. This second group of foods has an irritating effect on the esophageal lining. Spices can cause difficulties for some but not all people with heartburn. In all likelihood, the problem is that the spices are frequently used in recipes with high-fat or tomato-based sauces.

Depending on a person's tolerance, extremely hot or extremely cold food may act as an irritant. A way to test this might be to try eating foods or drinking beverages that are less intense on either side of the temperature scale. If the experiment works, it probably means that the esophagus was severely irritated. Finally, another group of beverages — beer, cola drinks, and milk — appears to be an offender by stimulating extra production of stomach acid.

By now, it's easy to see that a food diary is essential for controlling heartburn. It is important to write down everything you eat, and then note any distress you may experience. Try to pinpoint a specific food or ingredient if you can. Once you do, you should be able to develop your own personal list of foods to avoid and/or eliminate on a regular basis. Then, you can make changes that are suitable for you.

Try to keep in mind that large meals and bedtime or midnight snacks also promote heartburn. If at all possible, allow at least 2 to 3 hours from the last time you eat before going to bed, or even lying down for a nap. Heartburn will often occur if you tend to lie down after dinner to watch television — you're not letting gravity help move food downward. Planning small, frequent meals throughout the day is quite helpful in avoiding stomach distention.

Losing Weight For overweight individuals, here's another reason to lose weight. Excess pounds increase the pressure on your stomach, thus worsening reflux. Many people put food in their mouths almost as an unconscious habit, even when they don't feel hungry. It's helpful in this situation to follow some simple rules: Don't eat between meals. Dine at an unhurried pace — never swallow food until you've chewed it carefully.

The types of food to avoid when you're trying to lose weight are the same as those that have a harmful effect on LES — high-fat food, chocolate, and alcohol. Finally, complement your weight reduction measures with a regular exercise regimen.

Avoiding Certain Medications When you see a doctor for persistent heartburn, remember to bring along a list of the medications you're currently taking. Just like certain foods—drugs, such as theophylline and calcium channel blockers, which are used to treat high blood pressure (see page 133)—can weaken the LES. Other agents, like nonsteroidal anti-inflammatory drugs (NSAIDs) and potassium chloride, are harmful because they can irritate the esophageal lining. Your physician will be able to advise you about medications.

Other Lifestyle Changes If you experience nocturnal heartburn, one of the most effective means of relief is elevating the head of the bed by 4 to 6 inches. You can raise the top of the bed by placing blocks or bricks under the bed-head, or by inserting a foam wedge under your upper body when you sleep. Extra pillows and waterbeds are not a good idea for people with heartburn; neither elevates the chest enough to help gravity clear material from the esophagus to the stomach.

Try to break your cigarette smoking habit if you have one, or at least reduce the number of cigarettes that you smoke. The effect of smoking on reflux is not fully understood, but a number of motility factors appear to be affected by it.

Avoid wearing tight belts or tight pants; in general, wear looser-fitting clothes. This simple measure can reduce abdominal pressure on the LES, and that will help to reduce reflux.

Be Good to Your Gut

Drug Treatment   It is likely that everyone who has ever had heartburn has tried antacids for relief. Antacids work by neutralizing the acidity of stomach contents so they are less irritating when reflux occurs; some antacid preparations contain a substance called alginic acid which produces a foam that floats inside the stomach on top of the stomach chyme and acts as a barrier against reflux.

When heartburn persists despite continued antacid use, or when prolonged antacid use causes diarrhea or some other side effect, it's definitely time to see your physician. (Note that depending on which type of antacid is used, certain problems can arise. Magnesium-based antacids may be a problem for kidney patients because they lead to magnesium retention; while altered calcium metabolism may result from calcium antacids.)

After making a diagnosis of GERD, your physician will counsel you on the lifestyle recommendations we've discussed and probably prescribe any one of a number of different classes of drugs. Medications called histamine-2 (H^2)-receptor blockers or proton-pump inhibitors decrease stomach acid production, the latter very profoundly. The H^2-receptor blockers— namely, cimetidine (Tagamet®, famotidine (Pepcid®), nizatidine (Axid®), and ranitidine (Zantac®)—as well as proton-pump inhibitors, such as omeprazole (Prilosec®) and lansoprazole (Prevacid®), are effective in reducing symptoms of GERD and decreasing antacid use.

Recently, famotidine and cimetidine became available in over-the-counter preparations at lower-than-prescription doses for the treatment of heartburn.

Another class of medicines, called promotility agents, may be prescribed for GERD. Such agents as metoclopramide (Maxolon®, Octamide®, Reglan®) and cisapride (Propulsid®) work by strengthening various motility factors, including the LES and the gastric emptying rate. These medications make it easier for food to move down through the esophagus, and pass out of the stomach.

Summary

Your physician will explain what the most appropriate treatments are for you. You can help the treatments succeed by adhering to the lifestyle recommendations plus any drug regimen you may be given. Remember that these recommendations will be effective only if you follow them long-term—even after an improvement in symptoms. Once you discontinue them, your heartburn is likely to return.

In a 1995 Gallup survey, 34% of symptomatic individuals said they've made changes in their eating habits. Some 26% indicated that they eat smaller, more frequent meals. And 11% said they've turned down invitations because food might be served late at night. Clearly, Americans have become more informed about what causes their heartburn and are paying attention to lifestyle recommendations.

Drugs that Can Cause Symptoms of Gastroesophageal Reflux*

Anticholinergics
Calcium channel blockers
Nicotine
Progesterone
Tetracycline
Quinidine
Potassium chloride
Tricyclic antidepressants
Iron salts
Nonsteroidal anti-inflammatory drugs

---

* The mechanisms vary; some seem to be related to reducing the pressure of the lower esophageal sphincter, while others cause esophageal injury.

RECIPES

Home-Style Waffles

Pumpkin Soup

*All-in-One Salmon Platter Meal
with Mustard Sauce*

Roast Chicken with Couscous

Skillet Chicken and Noodles

Three-Mushroom Risotto

Garlic-Steamed Green Beans

Baked Potato Fans

Basil-Scented Mashed Potatoes

Angel Food Cake

Bananas Au Rum

Home-Style Waffles

Makes 4 servings

Nothing says "special" like home-made waffles—especially when they are lower in fat and cholesterol than regular or store-bought ones. And don't limit waffles to breakfast; they're great for lunch, brunch, dinner, and dessert. To make waffles like a "pro," be sure you follow the directions that came with your waffle maker.

2 cups reduced-fat baking mix

1 1/3 cups lactose-free low-fat (1%) milk

2 tablespoons canola oil

4 egg whites, *divided*

Preheat waffle maker according to manufacturer's directions.

In a medium bowl combine the baking mix, milk, oil, and 2 of the egg whites; stir until mixture is just blended but still slightly lumpy. In a small bowl beat the remaining egg whites with an electric mixer until stiff peaks form; fold into flour mixture. *Do not over mix.*

Be Good to Your Gut

Pour batter onto grids of a preheated waffle maker. (Spray with nonstick cooking spray if indicated in waffle maker directions). Close lid quickly; do not open during baking.

Bake until steaming stops, or according to manufacturer's directions. Remove waffle from grid. Bake remaining waffles.

TASTE TIP:

Top waffles with maple syrup, honey, fruit syrup, or fresh or canned fruit. Or for a more substantial meal, top with creamed vegetables, chicken, or seafood, as tolerated.

NUTRITION VALUES PER SERVING
Calories 108.4
Fat 7.6g
Cholesterol 3.2mg
Sodium 85.5mg
Protein 6.2g
Carbohydrates 4.2g
Fiber 0.0g

Pumpkin Soup

Makes 4 servings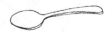

Pumpkin soup is delightfully versatile. A warm, hearty soup in the winter, it's also delicious served chilled in the summer. Canned pumpkin means that this soup is easy to prepare any time.

1 13 3/4-ounce can reduced-sodium chicken broth

1 16-ounce can solid pack pumpkin *(not pumpkin pie mix)*

2 tablespoons packed brown sugar

1/2 teaspoon ground ginger

1/4 teaspoon *each* ground cinnamon and salt

1/2 cup light sour cream

Toasted pumpkin seeds for garnish, *optional*

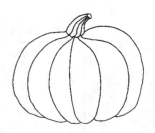

Be Good to Your Gut

In a medium saucepan stir together the broth, pumpkin, and *1/2 cup water* until smooth. Stir in the sugar, ginger, cinnamon, and salt. Bring just to a boil. Reduce heat, and simmer for 5 minutes, or until heated through. Remove from heat, and stir in the sour cream. Ladle the soup into bowls. Garnish with pumpkin seeds, if desired.

TASTE TIP:

Substitute 2 cups cooked, pureed butternut squash for the pumpkin, if desired. If soup is too thick, increase water slightly until thinned to desired consistency.

NUTRITION VALUES PER SERVING
Calories 103.5
Fat 2.5g
Cholesterol 3.2mg
Sodium 168.2mg
Protein 3.2g
Carbohydrates 18.2g
Fiber 3.3g

All-in-one Salmon Platter Meal with Mustard Sauce

Makes 4 servings

Here's a creative way to use your microwave oven. The entire meal is cooked at the same time, on the same plate. Fish is the perfect food for microwave cooking, and nothing could be easier. Use any fat-free salad dressing you tolerate well, and serve the mustard sauce on the side for the fish and potatoes.

3/4 pound Idaho potatoes *(about 2 medium), scrubbed, unpeeled, and cut in 1/4-inch slices*

1 1/4 pounds salmon fillets, *skinned and cut crosswise into four 1 1/2 x 3-inch pieces*

1 medium zucchini, *cut into 1-inch cubes*

1 medium red bell pepper, seeded and coarsely chopped

2 tablespoons fat-free salad dressing

1 cup fat-free sour cream

2 teaspoons *each* **fresh lemon juice and Dijon mustard, or to taste**

2 teaspoons chopped fresh herbs *(dill, tarragon, etc.)*

Arrange the potato slices in a single layer around the edge of a 12-inch round microwavable platter. Place the fish in a ring inside the potatoes. Mound the zucchini and pepper in the middle of the platter; sprinkle the dressing over the vegetables. Cover tightly with vented plastic wrap.

Microwave on HIGH for 8 to 10 minutes, or until the potatoes are tender, and the salmon is just cooked. Let stand for 3 minutes.

Meanwhile, in a small bowl whisk together the remaining ingredients with enough water (about 2 tablespoons) to thin to desired consistency. Serve with the salmon.

NUTRITION VALUES PER SERVING
Calories 335.2
Fat 9.6g
Cholesterol 77.0mg
Sodium 267.2mg
Protein 33.2g
Carbohydrates 26.9g
Fiber 2.6g

Roast Chicken with Couscous

Makes 6 servings

Whole-wheat couscous has a rich, nutty flavor. Look for it in the grain section of your supermarket, or in a health-food store. Left-over chicken can be used in the Oriental Chicken Soup (page 206), or your favorite chicken salad recipe.

10 ounces fresh spinach leaves, washed and coarsely chopped

2 cups cooked whole-wheat couscous

1/4 cup sliced almonds

2 tablespoons chopped fresh chives, optional

1/2 teaspoon dried dill weed

1/2 teaspoon salt

1 4 1/2 pound roasting chicken

Preheat oven to 350°F.

In a large nonstick skillet cook the spinach with *2 tablespoons water* over medium heat, tossing constantly, until just wilted. Drain well.

In a medium bowl stir together the spinach, couscous, almonds, chives (if using), dill, and salt; mix well.

Wash the chicken with cold water and pat dry. Remove any clumps of fat from inside the chicken. Stuff the chicken loosely with the couscous mixture. Tie the legs together using butcher's twine. Place chicken on a roasting rack in a roasting pan. Roast for about 2 hours, or until a meat thermometer inserted in the thickest part of the thigh meat registers 180°F. Remove the skin before serving.

TASTE TIP:

Let the chicken stand for about 15 minutes to make slicing easier. Fresh spinach can be replaced with a 10-ounce package of frozen spinach, thawed and well drained, if desired.

NUTRITION VALUES PER SERVING

Calories 463.5
Fat 17.1g
Cholesterol 163.5mg
Sodium 375.4mg
Protein 58.2g
Carbohydrates 17.1g
Fiber 2.0g

Be Good to Your Gut

Skillet Chicken and Noodles

Makes 4 servings

Here's a home-style recipe that is easy to fix and easy on your digestion. Just a touch of tomato paste blended with low-fat sour cream is easily tolerated for most people. Choose a good, sweet paprika for the best results. Hot cooked rice or boiled potatoes are also nice accompaniments to this dish.

1 cup reduced-sodium chicken broth

2 tablespoons tomato paste

2 tablespoons imported sweet paprika

1 teaspoon onion powder, optional

1 3-pound broiler chicken, cut into quarters

1 cup low-fat sour cream

2 tablespoons flour

1/4 teaspoon *each* salt and ground white pepper

1 cup thawed frozen baby peas

Hot cooked noodles

In a large nonstick frying pan combine the broth, tomato paste, paprika, and onion powder (if using); cook for 2 minutes, stirring occasionally.

Place the chicken in the pan skin side down. Cover, and reduce heat to low. Simmer for 20 minutes. Turn chicken pieces. Re-cover, and simmer 20 minutes longer, or until chicken is tender, and cooked through.

Remove the skin from the chicken, and transfer to a heated platter. Whisk in the sour cream, flour, salt, and pepper. Add the peas, and cook 2 minutes longer. Do not boil or sauce will curdle. Pour the sauce over the chicken and serve with the noodles.

TASTE TIP:

A finely chopped large tomato is a nice substitute for the tomato paste, if tolerated. The tomato loses much of its acidity when cooked, and the sour cream is a good buffer.

NUTRITION VALUES PER SERVING (*CHICKEN ONLY*)
Calories 473.3
Fat 17.9g
Cholesterol 163.5mg
Sodium 345.8mg
Protein 57.5g
Carbohydrates 16.7g
Fiber 1.5g

Three-Mushroom Risotto

Makes 4 servings

Domestic porcini, shitake, cremini… take
your pick of any three varieties of mushroom.
This recipe for risotto is easy to make. I like
to think of risotto as Italian comfort food, and
I think you'll agree with me on this one.
Using the pressure cooker makes it happen in
just about 5 minutes, or you can follow the
traditional hand-stirred method if you prefer.
The nice thing about using a pressure cooker
is that it seems to tame the onion, making it
less distressful than usual.

2 teaspoons extra-virgin olive oil

1 cup coarsely chopped onion

9 ounces mixed mushrooms, *any varieties,
cut into bite-size pieces*

1 1/2 cups Arborio *or* short-grain rice

3 1/2 to 4 cups mushroom stock *(page 20)
or reduced-sodium chicken broth*

1/4 cup chopped fresh basil

1/3 cup grated Parmesan cheese

Freshly ground black pepper, *optional*

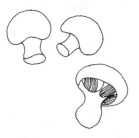

In a 6-quart pressure cooker heat the oil
over medium heat; stir in the onion and
cook for 1 minute. Stir in the mushrooms,
and cook 1 minute longer. Add the rice,
stirring to coat thoroughly with the oil. Stir
in 3 1/2 cups of the broth. Lock the lid in
place, and bring to high pressure over high
heat. Lower the heat just enough to maintain high pressure; cook 5 minutes longer.
Reduce pressure immediately, and remove
the lid, making sure to tilt it away from you
to allow excess steam to escape.

The risotto may be quite soupy although it
will continue to absorb liquid. If necessary
add a bit more broth. Stir in the basil, and
cheese, and ladle into shallow soup bowls.
Sprinkle with freshly ground black pepper,
if desired.

TASTE TIP:

*Substitute 1 teaspoon onion powder for the
onion, if desired. You may also stir in
some cooked chicken or fish at the end of
the cooking time.*

Stovetop Preparation:

In a large, heavy skillet, heat oil and follow directions up to the addition of broth. Add *1/2 cup of the broth*. Stir constantly until almost absorbed. Add the remaining broth, *1/2 cup at a time*, stirring constantly, until rice is al dente and the mixture is soupy. Stir in the basil, and the cheese, and serve as directed above.

NUTRITION VALUES PER SERVING

Calories 379.6
Fat 6.2g
Cholesterol 13.4mg
Sodium 216.9mg
Protein 12.2g
Carbohydrates 67.6g
Fiber 2.1g

Be Good to Your Gut

Garlic-Steamed Green Beans

Makes 4 servings

Steaming is probably the best way to cook green beans. It is effortless, and the beans come out crisp and flavorful. Sesame oil and sesame seeds are a lovely flavor boost for the beans as well. Since the garlic is only in the steaming water for flavor, it should be tolerable for everyone.

1 pound fresh green beans, *washed and trimmed*

1 cup water

1 clove garlic, *sliced*

2 teaspoons margarine *or* **soy margarine**

1/4 teaspoon dark sesame oil

1 tablespoon sesame seeds

In a small saucepan combine the water and garlic; bring to a boil. Place the beans in a steamer basket and place over, but not touching, the water. Cover, and reduce heat. Steam for 8 to 10 minutes, or until the beans are tender.

Transfer the beans to a serving dish. Add the remaining ingredients, and toss lightly until the beans are glistening and the sesame seeds are well distributed.

TASTE TIP:

Broccoli can be substituted for the beans, if tolerated. Steam broccoli stems first for about 5 minutes; add florets and steam 4 to 5 minutes longer.

NUTRITION VALUES PER SERVING

Calories 68.6
Fat 3.5g
Cholesterol 0.0mg
Sodium 36.4mg
Protein 2.7g
Carbohydrates 8.6g
Fiber 2.1g

Be Good to Your Gut

Baked Potato Fans

Makes 4 servings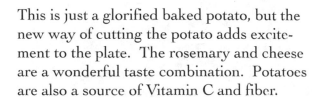

This is just a glorified baked potato, but the new way of cutting the potato adds excitement to the plate. The rosemary and cheese are a wonderful taste combination. Potatoes are also a source of Vitamin C and fiber.

4 medium Idaho potatoes, scrubbed

2 teaspoons canola oil

1 1/2 teaspoons fresh rosemary

2 tablespoons grated Parmesan cheese

Preheat oven to 400°F.

Place the potatoes, flat side down, on cutting board. Make four to five vertical cuts into the potato, three-quarters of the way through, forming a "fan." *Do not cut all the way through the potato*. Soak the potatoes for 15 to 20 minutes in ice water if time permits. Dry the potatoes, and rub with the oil. Sprinkle with the rosemary, and then with the cheese.

Place the potatoes on a baking sheet, and bake for 50 to 60 minutes, or until the potatoes are done, and the cheese is golden brown.

TASTE TIP:

Dried oregano or basil can be substituted for the rosemary, if desired.

NUTRITION VALUES PER SERVING
Calories 119.7
Fat 3.2g
Cholesterol 2.0mg
Sodium 53.3mg
Protein 3.4g
Carbohydrates 20.3g
Fiber 1.8g

Basil-Scented Mashed Potatoes

Makes 4 servings

Here is a dairy-free and cholesterol-free way to enjoy smooth mashed potatoes. You can even make these ahead of time and reheat in the microwave. When you do, sprinkle some water or broth over the top to keep them moist.

1 1/4 pounds Idaho potatoes, *peeled and quartered*

1 tablespoon olive oil

3 tablespoons finely chopped fresh basil, *or to taste*

1/2 teaspoon salt

1/8 teaspoon ground white pepper

In a large saucepan, place the potatoes and enough cold water to cover. Bring to a boil over high heat. Reduce heat, and simmer for about 12 to 15 minutes, or until the potatoes are tender. Drain and reserve cooking water.

Return the potatoes to the saucepan. Add the remaining ingredients. Using an electric mixer, mash the potatoes adding, enough of the reserved cooking water until the desired consistency is reached.

TASTE TIP:

Use fresh chives, tarragon, or another herb, if you like. When mashing potatoes, substitute chicken broth for the cooking water.

NUTRITION VALUES PER SERVING
Calories 142.5
Fat 3.5g
Cholesterol 0.0mg
Sodium 275.0mg
Protein 3.0g
Carbohydrates 25.6g
Fiber 2.3g

Be Good to Your Gut

Angel Food Cake

Makes 12 servings

Angel food cake is a dessert that everyone can appreciate. Light and delicious, this is a fat-free and cholesterol-free way to enjoy something sweet. Serve it on its own, or jazz it up with sliced fresh fruit, a fruit sauce, or even a bit of chocolate syrup drizzled on top, if you like.

Using a serrated bread knife is the best way to cut an angel food cake, unless you want to purchase a comb-like metal cake divider made just for this task.

1 cup superfine sugar, *divided*

1 cup minus 1 tablespoon sifted cake flour

10 large egg whites, *at room temperature*

3/4 teaspoon cream of tartar

1/4 teaspoon salt

1 1/2 teaspoons vanilla extract

1/2 teaspoon almond extract, *optional*

Preheat oven to 375°F.

In a medium bowl, whisk together *1/2 cup of the sugar*, and the cake flour; set aside.

In a large bowl using an electric mixer at medium speed, beat the egg whites until thick and foamy. Increase mixer speed to high; add the cream of tartar, salt, vanilla, and almond extract (if using). Continue beating until soft peaks form. Gradually sprinkle the remaining sugar over the top, and continue beating on high speed until peaks are glossy and stiff, but not dry and overbeaten.

Using a rubber spatula or slotted spoon, gently and quickly fold in the flour mixture in 3 batches. Pour into an *ungreased* 10-inch tube pan with removable sides; run a sharp knife through the batter to break up any air pockets.

Bake for 30 to 35 minutes, or until a tester inserted in the center of the cake comes out clean.

Hang the cake upside down on a wine bottle or funnel or invert on a wire rack, and cool completely. Run a thin metal spatula or sharp knife around the sides and release from pan.

NUTRITION VALUES PER SERVING

Calories 118.3
Fat 0.1g
Cholesterol 0.0mg
Sodium 106.5mg
Protein 3.7g
Carbohydrates 25.9g
Fiber 0.2g

Be Good to Your Gut

Bananas Au Rum

Makes 4 servings

Bananas don't need to be just for breakfast
and cereal anymore. Bananas are famous for
their high potassium content, as well as for
the fiber they contain. Orange, apple, or
apricot juice can be substituted for the rum, if
tolerated.

2 teaspoons margarine or soy margarine

1/4 cup packed dark brown sugar

1/4 cup dark rum

3 firm ripe bananas

Vanilla frozen yogurt, *optional*

In a large nonstick skillet heat the margarine over medium-high heat. Stir in the
brown sugar, and cook until dissolved. Stir
in the rum, and cook over low heat for 1
minute.

Peel the bananas, and cut in half horizontal-
ly; cut each half in half vertically. Place the
banana slices into the skillet with the rum

mixture. Cook over medium heat for 1 to 2
minutes, basting the bananas, until they are
heated through. Spoon into dessert dishes,
and top with frozen yogurt, if desired.

TASTE TIP:

*To reduce alcohol, combine 1/2 teaspoon
rum extract with 1/4 cup water as a substitute for the rum. A few tablespoons of
chopped dates add flavor and texture, if
desired.*

NUTRITION VALUES PER SERVING

Calories 162.4
Fat 2.4g
Cholesterol 0.0mg
Sodium 30.7mg
Protein 0.9g
Carbohydrates 28.8g
Fiber 1.4g

INDIGESTION

We're all familiar with the occasional upset stomach and indigestion after eating a meal. What most of us then do is reach for the antacid bottle in the medicine cabinet. When antacids and other over-the-counter remedies don't relieve the discomfort, or when these stomach complaints and accompanying symptoms—such as bloating and upper abdominal distress or even pain—worsen or occur troubling frequency, people turn to their doctors for help. About 5 percent of all visits to family physicians and other primary care practitioners are for indigestion, as are up to one-third of referrals to gastroenterologists.

Doctors have a name for indigestion: *dyspepsia*, which merely means bad digestion. People may not have all the symptoms of dyspepsia described here, but by and large they know when they have it. Doctors also feel that they know when they are seeing a case of dyspepsia. Experts have not agreed on a precise definition of the disorder, however. It is not surprising, then, that both primary care physicians and specialists find

the job of diagnosing and treating dyspepsia
a real challenge.

A recent survey indicated that 36 percent of adult Americans have indigestion.
More women than men suffer from indigestion, especially in their child-bearing
years. Individuals with indigestion typical-
ly will complain of some combination of
heartburn, regurgitation, belching, bloating, feeling full after eating even a small
meal, gassiness, nausea, and perhaps vomiting. Often, symptoms increase in frequency and the discomfort escalates. When
indigestion becomes chronic, it is a source
of constant pain in the middle- to-upper
part of the stomach.

These symptoms may resemble the complaints of a person with gastroesophageal
reflux disease (GERD), and it is true that
the two conditions are very similar.
Heartburn and regurgitation, in particular,
are common to both. Most symptoms clearly are related to eating. In addition, impair-
ment of GI motility — the underlying cause
of GERD — appears to be frequent in people with dyspepsia as well. Muscle contractions in the lower stomach after meals are
less frequent and weaker in dyspeptic than
in healthy individuals, and slowness in emptying food from the stomach (called gastroparesis) is a common finding.

Nevertheless, dyspepsia is a distinct condition from GERD. In many individuals,

GERD may be the cause of the dyspepsia, but other diseases also give rise to the same symptoms. These other possible diagnoses include peptic ulcers, gallstones, pancreatic disease, and, in rare instances, stomach cancer, to name a few. More often than not, though, people have unexplained dyspepsia. That is, there are no abnormalities on physical examination and the series of tests ordered by the doctor come back negative.

When diagnostic tests identify the underlying cause, the dyspepsia is said to have an organic origin. When there is no obvious cause, the dyspepsia is functional. Functional dyspepsia is made more difficult to recognize by the presence, in more than 1 in 3 people, of chronic *lower* abdominal pain and changes in bowel habits.

Whether or not someone's indigestion is caused by GERD, motility may still be an important contributing factor. In addition, diet has long been implicated in dyspepsia. For example, foods rich in fat stay in the stomach longer and may lead to delayed stomach emptying. Dyspeptic individuals may also be highly sensitive to stomach distention and thus quicker to feel pain at smaller degrees of stomach bloating. This may account for the onset of dyspeptic symptoms after eating. Some experts believe that emotional stress may result in dyspepsia, either directly or indirectly, by affecting stomach motility or by aggravating an irritable bowel.

When a person complains primarily of heartburn and regurgitation, the doctor may make a diagnosis of reflux disease, advise the person to adopt lifestyle changes that have positive effects on motility, and start him or her on medications to treat reflux. If there is no response to these measures, the possibility of dyspepsia should then be considered.

Patients with dyspepsia can help their doctors by describing their symptoms clearly and fully. For example, how severe is the nausea? How frequently does it occur? Is the pain sharp or dull or gnawing? How long have you had it? Does the symptom occur after eating or drinking certain foods, or after exercise? Is it related to a stressful event? In women, is it related to the menstrual cycle?

Your physician also should be informed of any medication that you are taking, because many commonly prescribed drugs can contribute to dyspeptic symptoms. Excessive intake of alcohol may also be the culprit.

Depending on the medical history and results of the physical examination as well as your age, any of a number of tests may be ordered. It is very likely to include a rectal stool examination and routine blood count to check for bleeding. Imaging of the upper and lower GI tract may be appropriate, whether by endoscopy or barium x-ray, to determine the presence or absence of peptic ulcer disease or malignancy. Because chest pain may indicate heart disease, an electro-cardiogram (ECG) or exercise stress test may be performed. If results are negative, many people will be relieved to learn that they do not have an ulcer or heart disease. Other possible tests include an ultrasound scan — possibly of the pancreas — or even a psychological evaluation.

The possibility that tests may reveal a serious illness suggests that dyspepsia is not always "simple." Recognizing and treating dyspepsia remains an important challenge for researchers and physicians alike.

What to Do about It

In patients with organic dyspepsia, the aim is to treat the underlying cause of the symptoms. With functional dyspepsia, the physician may recommend a therapeutic trial of medication. In both groups of patients, a few relatively simple dietary modifications may be effective. You may also want to see a registered dietitian for personalized nutrition counseling sessions. These meetings are especially useful in helping to get a clear picture of what you're currently eating. The dietitian will probably ask you to take along a record of what you've eaten for the past three days. With that information in hand, he or she will help you to identify particular patterns or foods that are related to your indigestion.

Diet If you suspect that your indigestion is caused by eating certain foods, a food diary in which you list every food and beverage consumed throughout the day is the best aid to help you establish a possible link. Be sure to write down everything.

Big family dinners, holiday parties, and social gatherings are all too often followed by indigestion. Smaller, more frequent meals are helpful for many people. You'll also probably feel more comfortable if you reduce or eliminate your intake of caffeine and alcohol. Remember that even decaffeinated beverages can cause indigestion in some people.

Specific foods that seem to provoke indigestion include orange juice, tomato juice, tomatoes, and radishes. Few people with indigestion complain of spices being a problem, but if your food diary shows a routine upset after you eat a certain herb or spice, by all means, eliminate it. Though some people think they are reacting to spicy sauces, it is more likely the tomato base of the sauce that is the problem—not the spice itself. A little trial and error on your part, along with notes in your food diary, will help you determine what is troublesome for you.

Keeping the fat content of meals and snacks low is a good idea. Remember that

162   *Be Good to Your Gut*

fat tends to slow down the rate at which the stomach empties. The less fat the stomach has to handle, the less time the food will be there. And the more quickly it moves to the next stage of digestion, the less likely it is to create a problem. There's no doubt that if stomach motility is slow, or if you eat large, fatty meals washed down with alcohol and coffee, indigestion is bound to be a problem. You might try eating less fried and greasy foods like fried chicken, french fries, heavy sauces, and gravy. Salad dressings and large portions of cheese and nuts should also be reduced. You may not have to eliminate any food at all. Just eating less of it could be the solution.

Stress Stress figures prominently in any discussion of indigestion. However, its exact role can be more elusive than that of dietary factors. For example, it becomes clear after a while that every time fried food is eaten, indigestion occurs. But the connection between a stressful work situation, for instance, and the incidence of belching or bloating is far less obvious. That's because we're often unaware that stress is present, or of the possible effects it may have.

One way to track stress is through your food diary. When making notes of what you're eating, also consider entering information such as where you were and whom you were with at the time. Note how you were feeling and what was happening in your life. If you are able to connect a particular event with stress (and the ensuing indigestion), the cause may be stress-related. In that case, see what you can do to deal with the person or circumstance causing the stress. Simply identifying the source may help you to eliminate it.

Habits such as not chewing thoroughly or eating too quickly can contribute to indigestion. Both of these habits may be stress reactions. Simple as it may sound, try to eat in a relaxed atmosphere. Of course, that's the tricky part. In all probability, to do that, you're going to have to adjust your schedule a bit—or the schedule of your family—to make things less hectic during mealtimes. When you do, you'll find it's well worth the effort.

Finally, refer to the section in the irritable bowel syndrome chapter (pages 84-85) in which techniques such as biofeedback and hypnosis are listed. They can be especially helpful if the indigestion is related to anxiety or to swallowing too much air.

Other Suggestions

Most sufferers of dyspepsia will have tried antacids, without long-term success, before paying their physician a visit. Recently, certain medications called histamine-2 (or H_2)-blockers—cimetidine

164

(Tagamet®) and famotidine (Pepcid®) —
became available in over-the-counter preparations to treat acid indigestion at
lower-than-prescription dosages.

Experience tells us that not all drugs used
to relieve dyspepsia will work for all individuals. Nevertheless, some people do feel better,
for instance with H_2-blockers at prescription
strengths. Success has also been reported
with a class of medications called the proki-
netics. These latter drugs — an example is cisapride (Propulsid®) — have beneficial effects
on the rate of stomach emptying.

Aspirin, aspirin-containing products,
ibuprofen, or other nonsteroidal anti-inflammatory drugs (NSAIDs) are definitely not
recommended to relieve any type of indigestion or related stomach pain. In fact, these
drugs, which many older people take for
arthritis and other conditions, can irritate
the lining of the stomach and cause injury.
An antacid preparation (Mylanta®) may be
particularly helpful in dyspepsia caused by
NSAID use.

Summary

For the most part, the best solutions for
coping with indigestion are based on com-
mon-sense advice about diet and lifestyle. A
therapeutic diet, in the strict sense, is rarely
necessary for most people. Eating a variety

of foods at regular intervals, lowering the fat content of what you eat, limiting consumption of alcohol and tobacco, moderating caffeine intake, and reducing levels of emotional stress are the best recommendations to follow.

When heartburn is a complaint, changes like elevating the head of the bed at night and reducing or stopping cigarette smoking altogether are also recommended (see page 123 for more suggestions).

When occasional bouts of indigestion occur with increasing frequency and become progressively more severe, it's time to see your physician for a thorough examination.

RECIPES

Honey Corn Muffins

Buttermilk Pancakes

Fish Chowder

Herb-Roasted Chicken

Beef Lo-Mein

Saffron Risotto with Scallops

Cheesy Squash and Potatoes

Sweet Potatoes with Pineapple

Peach-Cranberry Cobbler

Angel Kisses

Pumpkin Snack Cake

Honey Corn Muffins

Makes 12 muffins

Corn bread, corn sticks or corn muffins all taste great—especially in the morning. Each one can be made from this same recipe baked in different shaped pans.

1 cup all-purpose flour

1 cup yellow corn meal

4 teaspoons baking powder

1/2 teaspoon salt

1 cup low-fat (1%) lactose-free milk

1/4 cup thawed frozen egg substitute

3 tablespoons corn oil

2 tablespoons honey*

Preheat oven to 400°F. Lightly spray a muffin pan with nonstick cooking spray; set aside.

In a large bowl whisk together the flour, corn meal, baking powder, and salt. In a medium bowl or large measuring cup combine the milk, egg substitute, corn oil, and honey.

Be Good to Your Gut

Make a well in the center of the flour mixture. Pour in the milk mixture; stir until just combined. Spoon batter evenly into prepared pan. Bake for 18 to 22 minutes, or until golden brown. Transfer the muffins to a wire rack to cool.

*Measure the honey with the same tablespoon in which you measured the oil; the honey will slide easily into the bowl.

TASTE TIP:

White corn meal can be substituted for the yellow corn meal.

NUTRITION VALUES PER MUFFIN
Calories 138.4
Fat 4.3g
Cholesterol 0.8mg
Sodium 253.4mg
Protein 3.3g
Carbohydrates 22.2g
Fiber 2.2g

Buttermilk Pancakes

Makes 4 servings

Pancakes are quick and easy to prepare. They make breakfast a time to look forward to. Top them with your favorite syrup or canned or fresh fruit.

1 1/4 cups all-purpose flour

2 tablespoons sugar

1 teaspoon baking powder

1/2 teaspoon baking soda

1/4 teaspoon salt

1 1/3 cups low-fat buttermilk

1/4 cup thawed frozen egg substitute

1 tablespoon canola oil

In a medium bowl stir together the flour, sugar, baking powder, baking soda, and salt. In a small bowl combine the buttermilk, egg substitute, and oil. Add all at once to the flour mixture, stirring until just blended but still a bit lumpy. (Add additional buttermilk to thin the batter, if necessary.)

Be Good to Your Gut

Pour about 1/4 cup of the batter onto a hot, lightly oiled nonstick griddle or skillet. Cook for 1 to 2 minutes, or until pancakes have a bubbly surface and are slightly dry around the edges. Turn, and cook for 1 to 2 minutes longer, or until lightly browned.

TASTE TIP:

Drop 5 or 6 fresh blueberries onto pancakes just as they start to bubble. Or experiment with dried cranberries or cherries, if tolerated, stirred into the batter. (Let the batter stand for 3 to 5 minutes before cooking.)

NUTRITION VALUES PER SERVING
Calories 238.1
Fat 4.5g
Cholesterol 2.9mg
Sodium 456.0mg
Protein 8.5g
Carbohydrates 40.6g
Fiber 1.1g

Fish Chowder

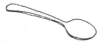

Makes 4 servings

There's nothing like a chowder chock full of potatoes and fish. Here's one that doesn't take hours to make. Leave the fish in one or two whole pieces until the soup is done. The fish will break up into nice bite-size chunks when you ladle it into bowls for serving.

2 teaspoons vegetable oil

1 cup chopped celery

2 cups diced potatoes

2 8-ounce bottles clam juice, *or* **water**

1 bay leaf

1/4 teaspoon dried thyme

1 cup lactose-reduced milk

1 pound cod fillets

Chopped fresh parsley for garnish, *optional*

In a medium saucepan heat the oil over medium heat. Stir in the celery, and potatoes; cook for 1 minute, stirring constantly. Add the clam juice, bay leaf, and thyme; cook over medium heat, uncovered, for 12 to 15 minutes, or until the potatoes are tender. Remove the bay leaf. Stir in the milk.

Be Good to Your Gut

Add the fish (in 1 or 2 whole pieces as described above); cook over low heat for about 5 minutes, or until fish is opaque and cooked through. Do not stir during cooking. Ladle the soup into serving bowls. Garnish with parsley, if desired.

TASTE TIP:

Flounder, scrod, or red snapper can be substituted for the cod. If tolerated, 1/4 teaspoon onion powder can be added.

NUTRITION VALUES PER SERVING
Calories 207.1
Fat 3.9g
Cholesterol 51.1mg
Sodium 371.6mg
Protein 24.6g
Carbohydrates 18.1g
Fiber 1.4g

Herb-Roasted Chicken

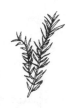

Makes 6 servings

Here's a wonderfully simple and aromatic
way to make chicken any night of the week.
If you have some leftover, use it in the
Country Vegetable-Bean Soup (page 52)
for a hearty meal.

1 **orange,** *washed and quartered*

1 **lemon,** *washed and quartered*

1 **tablespoon olive oil**

1 **4 1/2 pound roasting chicken**

Salt

3 **sprigs fresh rosemary** *or* **thyme** *(each
  about 2 1/2 inches long*

Preheat oven to 350°F.

Squeeze the juice from the orange and
lemon into a small bowl (saving the fruit).
Add the oil, and set aside.

Wash the chicken with cold water and pat
dry. Sprinkle the interior of the bird with
salt. Place as much of the reserved fruits as
will fit, and one sprig of the rosemary

inside. Gently slip your forefingers under the skin of the chicken at the neck opening, one at each side of the breast. Continue to work your fingers down the side of the breast to form a pocket. Insert one of the rosemary sprigs on each side. Tie the legs together using butcher's twine, if desired. Place the chicken on a roasting rack in a roasting pan. Roast for about 1 1/2 hours, or until a meat thermometer inserted in the thickest part of the thigh meat registers 180°F. Baste occasionally with the juice mixture. Remove the skin before serving.

TASTE TIP:

Let the chicken stand for about 15 minutes to make slicing easier. Any flavoring can be used inside the chicken and under the skin. Vegetables such as carrots and celery are good in the cavity. Mustards, jams, or sliced fruits can be slipped under the skin. Use pepper to season the interior of the cavity, if tolerated.

NUTRITION VALUES PER SERVING
Calories 249.4
Fat 9.2g
Cholesterol 109.0mg
Sodium 138.3mg
Protein 35.9g
Carbohydrates 5.2g
Fiber 0.8g

Beef Lo-Mein

Makes 4 servings

This low-fat, one-dish meal has something for everyone—lots of complex carbohydrates in the pasta, a bit of protein in the beef, and fiber in the vegetables.

6 ounces whole-wheat vermicelli

8 ounces round steak, *cut into thin strips*

1 cup reduced-sodium beef broth

3 tablespoons reduced-sodium soy sauce

2 tablespoons sherry wine

1 teaspoon sesame oil

1 teaspoon cornstarch

1/2 teaspoon sugar

2 cups bean sprouts

1 cup shredded carrots

1 cup thawed, frozen peas

1 8-ounce can sliced water chestnuts,
 drained

Bring 4 quarts of water to a boil; stir in the pasta. Cook for about 8 to 10 minutes, or until the pasta is al dente. Drain; and set aside.

Be Good to Your Gut

Spray a large nonstick skillet with cooking spray. Add the meat, and cook over medium-high heat for 3 to 5 minutes, or until done. Transfer the meat to a small dish, and wipe the skillet clean with a paper towel.

In a small bowl combine the broth, soy sauce, wine, and oil; stir in the cornstarch and sugar until dissolved. Pour the mixture into the skillet, and cook over medium heat for about 1 minute. Add the sprouts, carrots, peas, and water chestnuts. Cook for about 3 to 4 minutes, tossing lightly, until heated through. Stir in the pasta and meat; toss lightly until combined. Cook 2 minutes longer.

TASTE TIP:

Substitute linguine or thin spaghetti for the vermicelli.

NUTRITION VALUES PER SERVING
Calories 361.7
Fat 5.1g
Cholesterol 49.0mg
Sodium 492.1mg
Protein 30.2g
Carbohydrates 49.3g
Fiber 7.8g

Saffron Risotto with Scallops

Makes 4 servings

You can make perfect risotto in the pressure cooker in just 5 minutes. It's almost magic. This delicate version is a wonderful comfort food. Standard directions are also provided for those who prefer a conventional, hand-stirred version. If you're using canned broth, eliminate the salt.

2 teaspoons extra-virgin olive oil

1 cup thinly sliced leeks *(white and about 1 inch of the green part), rinsed thoroughly*

1 1/2 cups Arborio *or* short-grain rice

3 1/2 to 4 cups reduced-sodium vegetable *or* chicken broth

1/8 teaspoon saffron threads

1/4 cup chopped fresh Italian (flat-leaf) parsley

1/4 teaspoon salt

1/2 pound bay scallops

1/4 cup grated Asiago cheese

Freshly ground black pepper, optional

In a 6-quart pressure cooker heat the oil over medium heat; stir in the leeks and cook for 1 minute. Add the rice, stirring thoroughly to coat with the oil. Stir in 3 1/2 cups of the broth and the remaining ingredients, except the scallops, cheese, and pepper (if using). Lock the lid in place, and bring to high pressure over high heat.

Lower the heat just enough to maintain high pressure; cook 5 minutes longer. Reduce pressure immediately and remove the lid, making sure to tilt it away from you to allow excess steam to escape.

The risotto may be quite soupy (though it will continue to absorb liquid; if necessary, add a bit more broth). Stir in the scallops, and cheese; and cook over low heat until the scallops are just opaque, about 2 minutes. Ladle into shallow soup bowls. Sprinkle with freshly ground black pepper, if desired.

TASTE TIP:

Omit the leeks if they are a problem for you. Add 1 1/2 teaspoons onion powder instead, if tolerated. Toss in some cooked vegetables such as chopped spinach or carrot, if desired.

Stovetop Preparation:

In a large heavy skillet heat oil and follow directions up to the addition of broth. Add 1/2 cup of the broth, and stir constantly until almost absorbed. Add remaining broth, 1/2 cup at a time, stirring constantly, until the rice is al dente and the mixture is soupy. Stir in the scallops, and cheese and serve as directed above.

NUTRITION VALUES PER SERVING
Calories 374.3
Fat 6.6g
Cholesterol 44.6mg
Sodium 388.7mg
Protein 23.1g
Carbohydrates 57.1g
Fiber 3.1g

Cheesy Squash and Potatoes

Makes 4 servings

Simply combining two of your favorites can add new interest to your menu. This very delightful side dish will do just that.

3/4 pound Idaho potatoes, *peeled and quartered*

3/4 pound butternut squash, peeled, *seeded, and cut into 2-inch chunks*

1/2 cup shredded Swiss cheese (2 ounces)

1 tablespoon chopped pecans for garnish

In a medium saucepan cover the potatoes and squash with cold water, and bring to a boil. Cook over medium heat for about 20 minutes, or until tender. Drain well, and return to saucepan; add the cheese. Using a vegetable masher or electric mixer, mash until smooth and well blended. Garnish with nuts and serve.

TASTE TIP:

Two tablespoons of whipped low-fat cream cheese or cottage cheese can be substituted for the Swiss cheese, if desired.

NUTRITION VALUES PER SERVING

Calories 163.9
Fat 5.2g
Cholesterol 13.0mg
Sodium 44.7mg
Protein 6.6g
Carbohydrates 24.4g
Fiber 3.2g

Sweet Potatoes with Pineapple

Makes 4 servings

Sweet potatoes add new flavor and bright color to any meal. They're also a good source of beta-carotene. Serve this delightful side dish with Herb-Roasted Chicken (page 176); it's a winning combination.

4 medium sweet potatoes, *scrubbed*

1 cup canned crushed pineapple *(packed in juice), drained*

2 tablespoons margarine *or* soy margarine

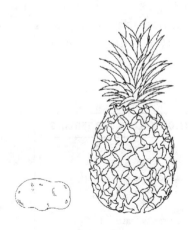

Preheat oven to 375°F.

Bake the sweet potatoes for 50 to 60 minutes, or until tender. When potatoes are cool enough to handle, cut a lengthwise slice from the top of each potato. Scrape the potato into a medium bowl, reserving the hollowed-out skins.

Use an electric mixer or vegetable masher to mash the potatoes well; stir in the pineapple and margarine until blended. Spoon the mixture back into the potato skins. Place the potatoes on a baking sheet, and reheat for 5 to 10 minutes, if desired.

NUTRITION VALUES PER SERVING
Calories 237.4
Fat 6.5g
Cholesterol 0.0mg
Sodium 98.4mg
Protein 2.5g
Carbohydrates 44.4g
Fiber 3.2g

Peach-Cranberry Cobbler

Makes 8 servings

Fruit cobblers are a wonderful dessert any time of the year. Use fresh fruits when they're in season or canned ones whenever you're in the mood for a warm, homemade treat.

4 cups canned sliced peaches *(packed in juice), drained, and liquid reserved*

1/4 cup packed brown sugar, *divided*

4 teaspoons cornstarch

1 cup reduced-fat baking mix

1/4 cup low-fat (1%) lactose-free milk

1 tablespoon vegetable oil

1/4 cup dried cranberries

1/2 teaspoon grated lemon rind

Preheat oven to 425°F. Lightly spray an 8-inch square baking pan with nonstick cooking spray; set aside.

In a medium saucepan combine 1/2 cup of the reserved peach liquid, 3 tablespoons of the sugar, and the cornstarch until blended. Cook over low heat, stirring constantly, until bubbly and thickened; stir in the peaches, and set aside.

In a small bowl stir together the baking mix, milk, oil, cranberries, and lemon rind until just combined. Pour the fruit mixture into the prepared pan and drop heaping table-spoons of the flour mixture on top. Bake for 15 to 18 minutes, or until top is golden brown. Transfer the pan to a wire rack to cool slightly. Serve warm.

TASTE TIP:

Peel and slice enough fresh peaches to make 4 cups of fruit, and substitute water or peach nectar for the peach liquid. Raisins or dried cherries can be substituted for the cranberries.

NUTRITION VALUES PER SERVING
Calories 126.0
Fat 2.2g
Cholesterol 0.3mg
Sodium 184.5mg
Protein 1.9g
Carbohydrates 25.4g
Fiber 2.7g

Be Good to Your Gut

Angel Kisses

Makes 20 cookies

These light meringue cookies practically melt in your mouth. Use egg whites that are at room temperature to guarantee full volume. Don't overbeat them, or the cookies will tend to dry out.

2 large egg whites at room temperature
Pinch cream of tartar, *optional*
1/3 cup superfine sugar
3/4 teaspoon vanilla extract

Preheat oven to 275°F. Spray a large cookie sheet with nonstick cooking spray, or line with a piece of baking parchment; set aside.

In a medium bowl using an electric mixer on medium speed, beat the egg whites until frothy. Add the cream of tartar (if using) and vanilla and beat on high speed, adding the sugar 1 tablespoon at a time, until the egg whites hold stiff peaks. Drop the batter by heaping teaspoons 2 inches apart onto the prepared cookie sheet. Bake for 25 minutes, or until cookies are golden, and the centers are set. Let cool on the sheet

for a few minutes. Transfer the cookies to a
wire rack to finish cooling. Store in a cool,
dry place.

TASTE TIP:

*Substitute almond or maple extract for
the vanilla, and stir in mini chocolate bits,
or finely chopped nuts, as tolerated.*

NUTRITION VALUES PER COOKIE
Calories 14.6
Fat 0.0g
Cholesterol 0.0mg
Sodium 7.1mg
Protein 0.4g
Carbohydrates 3.4g
Fiber 0.0g

Pumpkin Snack Cake

Makes 8 servings

Sometimes it's nice to have a snack that's flavorful but not too sweet. This moist cake does the trick. It's also nice with a sprinkling of confectioners' sugar, or topped with your favorite frosting.

1 1/2 cups all-purpose flour

1 teaspoon ground ginger

1/2 teaspoon *each* baking powder and baking soda

1/4 cup margarine *or* soy margarine

1/4 cup packed brown sugar

1/2 cup molasses

1/2 cup canned solid pack pumpkin (*not pumpkin pie mix*)

1/2 cup low-fat buttermilk

1/2 cup thawed frozen egg substitute

1 teaspoon vanilla extract

1/2 cup raisins

1 teaspoon grated orange rind

Preheat oven to 350ºF. Lightly spray an 8-inch square baking pan with nonstick cooking spray; set aside.

In a small bowl stir together the flour, ginger, baking powder, and baking soda. In a large bowl using an electric mixer, beat together the margarine, and sugar until blended. Add the molasses, pumpkin, buttermilk, egg substitute, and vanilla; beat on low speed until just blended. Stir in the flour mixture by hand until thoroughly combined. Fold in the raisins, and orange rind. Pour the batter into the prepared pan. Bake for 30 to 35 minutes, or until a cake tester inserted in the center of the cake comes out dry. Transfer the pan to a wire rack to cool.

TASTE TIP:

Chopped dates can be substituted for raisins, as dried cranberries or cherries. Add some chopped nuts, if tolerated.

NUTRITION VALUES PER SERVING
Calories 251.1
Fat 6.2g
Cholesterol 0.5mg
Sodium 223.6mg
Protein 5.2g
Carbohydrates 43.9g
Fiber 1.6g

Be Good to Your Gut

SLOW STOMACH EMPTYING (GASTROPARESIS)

If you've read the chapters on heart-burn and indigestion (see pages 119-129 and 157-166), you're already acquainted with the problem of slow stomach empty-ing. It involves a delay in the passage of food from the stomach into the small intes-tine, where the next stage of digestion takes place.

As a result of the delay in emptying, called gastroparesis, afflicted individuals may experience a host of unpleasant symp-toms. Many report feeling full after eating small meals or even a portion of a meal. Nausea immediately after eating and "dry heaves" may occur. Some people complain that they are able to taste food on their breath that they ate two or three days earli-er. Sometimes there is upper abdominal dis-comfort, pain, bloating, and vomiting. In severe cases, there may be substantial weight loss.

Gastroparesis can be the cause of these symptoms in patients with indigestion or gastroesophageal reflux disease. It is less well known that the same disorder can develop in diabetics. Let's look at the two types of diabetes mellitus: Type I (or insulin-dependent) diabetics produce no insulin, an important hormone for regulating blood sugar levels. Type II (non-insulin-dependent) diabetics produce an insufficient amount of insulin; they frequently overeat and are overweight.

Anywhere from 27 to 45 percent of people with type I diabetes are gastroparetic. Slow stomach emptying also occurs in type II diabetics. Although some people with gastroparesis do not complain of having symptoms, one report showed that as many as 76 percent of the diabetic population studied complained of early fullness, nausea, vomiting, and other symptoms.

Slow stomach emptying is a *motility* problem. That means there's something wrong with either the muscles that churn stomach contents, make smaller particles of ingested food, and then move it along the digestive tract, or with the nerves that trigger these muscles to expand and contract. In diabetics, the cause of gastroparesis is a complication called autonomic neuropathy.

The nerves making up the autonomic, or involuntary, nervous system control important bodily functions without any conscious direction. Thus, the heart beats on a constant, regular basis even though no "command" has been sent by the brain. This autonomic nervous system also controls the blood vessels, lungs, digestive tract, and bladder. Damage to the autonomic nerve (*autonomic neuropathy*) that triggers contraction of the stomach muscles may result in a slower rate of stomach emptying.

There are important reasons for identifying gastroparesis even in individuals who do not complain of symptoms. First, the gastroparesis can interfere with the diabetic's ability to control his or her blood sugar levels. These levels begin to fluctuate up and down in a way unrelated to the timing or dose of insulin. What isn't immediately evident to the diabetic is that food is staying in the stomach longer than usual, and then perhaps is suddenly pushed out. This disorder of stomach motility translates into a highly unpredictable rate of digestion and food absorption, which, in turn, produces wide swings in glucose levels and makes the insulin appear ineffective. But the reality is that the food has not yet moved far enough along the digestive tract for the insulin to do its job. Then, by the time the digested food leaves the stomach, the insulin has dissipated.

Sudden episodes of unexplained hyperglycemia (high blood glucose levels) or hypoglycemia (low levels) in a diabetic who previously had good blood glucose control is an important clue that gastroparesis may be present. Erratic blood glucose levels may be particularly evident in the morning.

Diabetics may fall into a harmful cycle in which gastroparesis results in high blood glucose levels, which then further slows the emptying of food from the stomach. Now, the diabetes is poorly controlled, and the gastroparesis worsens.

Not only are diabetics with autonomic neuropathy at risk for developing the symptoms of gastroparesis, but the onset of gastroparesis may also be an indication that their disease is progressing and that other serious complications of diabetes may follow. A diabetic with autonomic neuropathy may have diarrhea or, more frequently, constipation. Nerves in the urinary system may be damaged, resulting in weak muscle control and possibly incontinence.

These diabetics may experience palpitations or a pounding of the heart—a sure sign of tachycardia, or increased heart rate resulting from damage to heart nerves. They may get dizzy on standing up suddenly—a consequence of temporary low blood pressure due to nerve damage to the cardiovascular system. It is likely that diabetics with neuropathy also have disorders of the retina and of the kidney.

As diabetic neuropathy intensifies, the symptoms described earlier appear with greater frequency and severity. Occasionally when food (especially the fibrous parts of

194

plants) remains in the stomach too long, clumped stringy masses known as bezoars may form. These bezoars cause nausea, vomiting, and a sensation of blockage in the stomach. Foods such as oranges, coconuts, apples, figs, Brussels sprouts, green beans, potato skins, and sauerkraut commonly form bezoars. If your physician has indicated that you have this problem, it's important to avoid these foods.

The bottom line for diabetics: be aware of unexplained lapses in blood glucose control, and be sure to inform your physician when you have symptoms suggestive of slow stomach emptying.

What to Do About It

Controlling blood sugar is the overriding treatment goal for diabetics. When gastroparesis is present, in both diabetics and nondiabetics, efforts should be directed at relieving the symptoms. Diet is the first line of treatment. In addition, several medications with promotility effects are useful.

Diet Dietary recommendations are quite specific and usually not difficult to follow. Soft meals that are low in fat and fiber are encouraged. Because fat is known to slow gastric emptying, the total fat content in the diet should be reduced. Therefore, heavy sauces, baked goods, creamy or oily salad dressings, and fat-rich meats should definitely be limited.

On the other hand, proteins, complex carbohydrates such as cereals, fruits, and vegetables are usually permitted, but individual tolerance for these foods is the best guide. Most of the time, the dietary plan for gastroparesis can include a wide variety of popular foods. Lean meats, poultry, and fish, along with pasta, rice, and bread definitely stay on the menu. Sometimes, additional liquids or nutritional supplements may be added to the diet. That means more soups and juices, and perhaps a commercially prepared formula.

Often, smaller meals eaten more frequently throughout the day will help reduce the feeling of fullness and bloating. It is important to eat slowly and to chew foods thoroughly.

Severe cases of gastroparesis normally require a low-residue diet. For the most part, that means a low-fiber diet because foods containing plant fiber tend to stay longer in the stomach. Such a diet may be used only for a short time, the length depending on the severity of the motility problem and on the individual's tolerance for different foods.

Whole grains and whole-grain cereals, breads, nuts, seeds, and popcorn are definitely to be avoided in acute cases of gastroparesis. Legumes (beans and lentils), potatoes, all vegetables and fruits — canned as

196

well as fresh — also should be restricted in severe situations. Except for prune juice, fruit and vegetable juices are permitted. Even though milk and the connective tissue of some meat and shellfish are low in fiber, they still contribute to stool volume and thus should be avoided in serious cases of gastroparesis. For less severe cases, milk is limited to 2 cups a day. That limit includes the amount of milk in milk-based products such as ice cream and creamed soups.

Few people will need such strict limitations on their diets. However, those who do should find a good deal of relief from their discomfort when they follow the low-residue diet.

Avoiding Certain Medications Drugs including antidepressants, progesterone, and dopamine compounds used to treat Parkinson's disease can cause delayed stomach emptying (see page 198). It is important to inform your physician of any medication you're taking; some may impair stomach motility.

Drug Treatment

A number of medications accelerate stomach emptying and relieve associated symptoms. The prototype of these "promotility" drugs is metoclopramide (Maxolon®,

> ### _Drugs that May Cause Gastroparesis_
>
> _Anticholinergics_
> _Tricyclic antidepressants_
> _Opiates_
> _Progesterone_
> _Nicotine_
> _Alcohol_
> _Aluminum-containing antacids_

Octamide®, Reglan®), which is also useful in treating vomiting. However, side effects, including depression, drowsiness, and lethargy in about 20 percent of people taking metoclopramide limit its use. An investigational drug called domperidone (Motilium®) may be similarly effective, but without the side-effects profile of metoclopramide. Cisapride (Propulsid®) has no effect on vomiting, but otherwise has been shown to alleviate symptoms of gastroparesis. A frequently-used antibiotic, erythromycin (E-mycin®, Ilotycin®, Ethril®, and others), can stimulate gastrointestinal contractions and also may be useful in diabetic gastroparesis.

Summary

Managing diabetes requires a multidimensional approach. When gastroparesis is diagnosed, most diabetics will find it helpful to see a registered dietitian. A dietitian in the area may be recommended by the primary care physician. Many dietitians have advanced, specialized credentials; some may be certified diabetes educators (CDE). These individuals can be especially supportive to people with gastroparesis.

The good news is that more attention than ever is being paid to gastroparesis. With a combination of careful monitoring, diet, and perhaps medication, individuals with this condition can feel a lot more comfortable than in the past.

RECIPES

Maple Farina

Baked French Toast

Oriental Chicken Soup

Asian Rice Noodles with Chicken

Savory Steamed Fish

Couscous Sautéed with Orange Scallops

Carrot and Sweet Potato Puree

Creamy Cheesy Orzo

Peach Shortcakes

Home-Style Rice Pudding

Maple Farina

Makes 4 servings

Here's a fun way to add a wholesome and nutritious start to the day. For added fiber, sprinkle some toasted wheat germ over the cereal.

3 1/2 cups water

1/2 teaspoon salt

2/3 cup farina wheat cereal

4 tablespoons light maple syrup

4 canned pear halves, *drained and sliced*

Nonfat plain yogurt for garnish, *optional*

In a medium saucepan bring the water and salt to a boil. Reduce heat, and slowly pour the cereal into the water, stirring constantly. Cook for about 2 minutes, stirring constantly, until the cereal has thickened. Spoon cereal evenly into serving dishes. Drizzle each with 1 tablespoon of the syrup and top with the sliced pears. Garnish with yogurt, if desired.

TASTE TIP:

Substitute canned peaches, fruit cocktail, or apricots for the pears.

NUTRITION VALUES PER SERVING

Calories 206
Fat 0.3g
Cholesterol 0.0mg
Sodium 271.1mg
Protein 3.4g
Carbohydrates 48.3g
Fiber 2.8g

Baked French Toast

Makes 4 servings

This French toast only needs a fruit compote and a delicious cup of herbal tea to
accompany it to make an elegant brunch.
This recipe calls for soaking the bread the
night before, and then it's ready to bake as
your guests arrive.

1 cup low-fat (1%) lactose-free milk

1 cup thawed frozen egg substitute

1/4 cup sugar

1/2 teaspoon vanilla extract

**2 tablespoons Grand Marnier or
  orange juice**

8 thick slices French or sourdough bread
  (about 1 1/4-inches each)

Confectioners' sugar, *optional*

In a small bowl combine the milk, egg substitute, sugar, vanilla, and Grand Marnier
(or orange juice). In a large pan place the
bread in a single layer, and pour the milk
mixture over the top. Cover, and refrigerate
overnight, or for at least 5 hours.

Preheat oven to 400°F. Spray a baking sheet with nonstick cooking spray.

Transfer the bread to the baking sheet. Bake for 18 to 22 minutes, or until the bread is puffed and golden brown. Sprinkle lightly with confectioners' sugar before serving, if desired.

TASTE TIP:

Almond or coffee-flavored liqueurs are other variations to try. Or, top the French toast with a fruit-flavored syrup, fresh fruit such as crushed and sweetened strawberries or raspberries, or your favorite honey.

NUTRITION VALUES PER SERVING
Calories 382
Cholesterol 5.0mg
Sodium 653.0mg
Protein 17.0g
Carbohydrates 67.8g
Fiber 0.2g

Oriental Chicken Soup

Makes 4 servings

Simple and comforting, this Chinese-style soup is good as an appetizer. You can double the ingredients and serve in larger portions as an entree with crispy whole-wheat rolls.

1 13 3/4-ounce can reduced-sodium chicken broth

1 cup shredded cooked chicken

1 cup coarsely chopped fresh watercress

1 teaspoon reduced-sodium soy sauce

In a medium saucepan combine all the ingredients. Bring to a boil. Reduce heat, and simmer, uncovered, for 3 to 4 minutes, or until the watercress is slightly wilted.

TASTE TIP:
For a heartier soup, stir in 1 cup of cooked pasta or rice.

NUTRITION VALUES PER SERVING
Calories 82
Fat 1.9g
Cholesterol 39.6mg
Sodium 123.2mg
Protein 14.5g
Carbohydrates 0.9g
Fiber 0.1g

Be Good to Your Gut

Asian Rice Noodles with Chicken

Makes 4 servings

Rice noodles, found in Asian markets, blend well with any flavoring. They're soft, pleasant, and easy to digest. Substitute your favorite fish for the chicken, or add some additional cooked vegetables. This can be a vegetarian dish if you use vegetable broth and some tofu.

8 ounces 1/4-inch dried rice noodles

1/2 cup reduced-sodium chicken broth

4 teaspoons fish sauce* or low-sodium soy sauce, or to taste

1 teaspoon *each* sugar and paprika

1 1/2 teaspoons sesame oil

2 teaspoons grated ginger root

1 1/2 cups grated carrot

8 ounces cooked chicken, shredded

1/4 cup chopped fresh cilantro

In a large saucepan bring 2 quarts of water to a boil. Stir in the noodles, and cook for 30 seconds. Remove from heat, and let the noodles stand for 5 minutes, or until just firm. Drain.

In a measuring cup stir together the broth, fish sauce, sugar, and paprika; set aside.

In a large nonstick skillet heat the oil over medium heat. Stir in the ginger, and cook for 1 minute. Add the reserved broth mixture, and cook 1 minute longer. Add the remaining ingredients and the rice noodles. Stir 1 to 2 minutes, or until the noodles are heated through. Serve immediately.

TASTE TIP:

Substitute chili oil for the sesame oil for a livelier—and hotter—flavor, if tolerated. Garnish with 1/4 cup fresh shredded basil leaves.

NUTRITION VALUES PER SERVING

Calories 250
Fat 4.0g
Cholesterol 48.2mg
Sodium 811.5mg
Protein 19.8g
Carbohydrates 31.9g
Fiber 1.7g

Be Good to Your Gut

Savory Steamed Fish

Makes 4 servings

You can use a Chinese bamboo steamer, a wok, or a collapsible vegetable steamer placed in a deep skillet to cook this simple dish. If your wok doesn't have a steaming rack, place two wooden chopsticks (inside the wok) about 2 inches apart, and put a heatproof plate on top.

1 whole flounder, *or* **red snapper,** *or other lean white fish (about 2 1/2 pounds), scaled and cleaned, with head and tail removed*

2 large garlic cloves, *peeled and cut in half*

1 1/2 teaspoons dried rosemary

1 teaspoon dried thyme

2 tablespoons dry vermouth

Rinse the fish with cold water and pat dry; make 2 light slashes on each side with a sharp knife. Place the garlic inside the fish, and sprinkle the cavity with the rosemary and thyme.

Place the fish on a plate that will fit on a steamer rack. Sprinkle the vermouth over the fish.

Add about 2 inches of water to the steamer; bring to a boil. Place the plate on a rack (you may need to cut the fish in half if it doesn't fit in the steamer). Cover the steamer tightly, and steam the fish for about 12 minutes, or until the fish is opaque and flakes with a fork. Transfer to a serving platter. Remove the bones, and serve immediately with some of the accumulated juices spooned over the top.

TASTE TIP:

Use any of your favorite herbs in this recipe. Fresh basil leaves, tarragon, cilantro and parsley are good choices.

```
NUTRITION VALUES PER SERVING
        Calories 258
         Fat 2.1g
    Cholesterol 159.6mg
      Sodium 191.6mg
       Protein 53.2g
   Carbohydrates 1.6g
        Fiber  0.2g
```

Be Good to Your Gut

Couscous Sautéed with Orange Scallops

Makes 4 servings

When you're in the mood for a delicately-flavored dish but don't want to spend a lot of time cooking, this is the one to try. Couscous is easy to digest and versatile as can be. Substitute thin strips of chicken for the scallops if you prefer.

1 1/2 cups couscous

1 3/4 cups reduced-sodium chicken broth

1/4 teaspoon salt

2 teaspoons olive oil

10 ounces bay scallops, *peeled and deveined*

1 teaspoon grated orange peel

3 tablespoons orange juice

2 tablespoons chopped fresh parsley

In a medium bowl combine the couscous, broth, and salt. Cover, and set aside for 5 minutes.

Meanwhile, in a large nonstick skillet, heat the oil over medium-high heat. Add the scallops, and cook for 2 minutes. Add the orange peel, and cook 1 minute longer, or until the scallops are done. Remove from heat; stir in the orange juice and parsley.

Mound the couscous on a serving platter; spoon the scallops and pan juices over the top.

NUTRITION VALUES PER SERVING

Calories 375
Fat 4.1g
Cholesterol 41.1mg
Sodium 358.7mg
Protein 26.4g
Carbohydrates 57.9g
Fiber 1.1g

Carrot and Sweet Potato Puree

Makes 4 servings

How do you improve carrots or sweet potatoes? Combine them as a wonderful puree. You'll get cheers every time.

1 large sweet potato (about 8 ounces), *peeled and cut into 1/2-inch cubes*

1/2 pound carrots, *scraped and sliced*

1 tablespoon margarine or soy margarine

In a medium saucepan cover the sweet potatoes and carrots with cold water and bring to a boil. Cover and cook over medium heat for 15 to 20 minutes, or until tender.

Transfer the vegetables to a food processor. Add the margarine, and puree until smooth. (Alternately, use an electric mixer or vegetable masher to mash until smooth.)

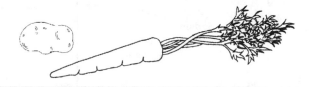

TASTE TIP:

Add 1/4 cup drained crushed pineapple and a dash of cinnamon or 1 tablespoon of sherry wine before mashing.

NOTE: Those on a very low-residue diet may not tolerate this recipe, or should have very small servings.

NUTRITION VALUES PER SERVING
Calories 110
Fat 3.3g
Cholesterol 0.0mg
Sodium 67.7mg
Protein 1.5g
Carbohydrates 19.5g
Fiber 3.5g

Be Good to Your Gut

Creamy Cheesy Orzo

Makes 4 servings

If you haven't discovered orzo yet, you're in for a wonderful surprise. Orzo is a tiny pasta that resembles rice, and it cooks in only 5 to 8 minutes. You'll find it in the pasta section of your local supermarket.

1 cup orzo

1/2 cup light sour cream

1/4 cup grated Parmesan cheese

2 tablespoons chopped fresh parsley

1/2 teaspoon salt

1 tablespoon chopped fresh chives for garnish

In a large saucepan bring 3 quarts of water to a boil; stir in the orzo. Reduce heat, and cook for 5 to 8 minutes, or until just tender. Do not overcook. Drain well. Transfer the orzo to a medium serving dish. Stir in the sour cream, cheese, parsley, and salt, mixing well to combine. Garnish with chives, and serve.

TASTE TIP:

Substitute 2 tablespoons margarine for the sour cream for a lighter version of this side dish.

NUTRITION VALUES PER SERVING
Calories 210
Fat 4.4g
Cholesterol 4.8mg
Sodium 403.8mg
Protein 8.3g
Carbohydrates 32.9g
Fiber 1.2g

Peach Shortcakes

Makes 4 servings

Serve this delicious dessert in every season. Use canned peaches in winter and fresh peaches in summer. Drizzle a little chocolate syrup over the top for an added treat.

1 16-ounce can sliced peaches packed in juice, drained *or 3 medium fresh peaches (about 2 cups sliced)*

1/2 teaspoon almond extract

4 prepared sponge cake shells

Thawed, frozen nondairy whipped topping and sliced almonds, for garnish

In a small bowl combine the peaches and almond extract. Cover, and chill until ready to serve.

Spoon the peaches into the shells. Garnish with the whipped topping and almonds.

NUTRITION VALUES PER SERVING
Calories 151
Fat 5.3g
Cholesterol 69.9mg
Sodium 53.8mg
Protein 2.7g
Carbohydrates 24.1g
Fiber 1.2g

Home-Style Rice Pudding

Makes 4 servings

There is nothing like home-made rice pudding to bring on feelings of warmth, comfort, and care. This low-fat, low-calorie version of an old favorite is sure to be a regular feature at your home.

2 1/2 cups low-fat (1%) lactose-free milk

1/2 cup uncooked rice

1/2 cup golden raisins

1/4 cup sugar

1/2 cup thawed frozen egg substitute

1/2 teaspoon vanilla extract

Ground cinnamon, *optional*

In a heavy medium saucepan bring the milk to just below a boil; reduce heat to low. Do not allow milk to boil. Stir in the rice, raisins, and sugar. Cover, and cook over low heat, stirring frequently, for 15 to 20 minutes, or until the rice is tender, and most of the milk is absorbed. Remove from the heat, and stir in the egg substitute and

Be Good to Your Gut

vanilla until mixture is smooth and creamy.
Spoon the pudding into dessert glasses and
sprinkle lightly with cinnamon, if desired.
Serve warm or chilled.

NOTE: Very low residue diets restrict milk
intake to less than 2 cups per day. Each
serving here contains about 1/2 cup.
Include this as tolerated.

NUTRITION VALUES PER SERVING

Calories 281
Fat 1.8g
Cholesterol 6.0mg
Sodium 140.8mg
Protein 11.8g
Carbohydrates 55.6g
Fiber 1.1g

A NEW LOOK AT LACTOSE

Lactose intolerance has been described as "the hot disorder of the 90s." According to some product advertisements, over 50 million Americans suffer from this disorder. If you think you are one of them, or if you are considering reducing or eliminating your intake of dairy products, read this chapter before you do anything rash. Remember that dairy products are an important source of several nutrients, including high-quality protein, phosphorus, potassium, magnesium and, of course, calcium.

Nutritionists and other health professionals can't stress enough the benefits of calcium. Here's why. In addition to serving as the major mineral component of bones and teeth, calcium regulates muscle contraction and relaxation, including that of the major muscle of the body: the heart. Calcium activates enzymes that are important in a variety of metabolic functions, and is needed for blood clotting. Because calcium is so vital for maintaining good health and a strong body structure, it is important to eat calcium-rich foods every day.

One reason people skimp on calcium-rich foods is a concern about lactose intolerance. Some reports estimate that 28 percent of American adults have a limited ability to fully digest lactose, the sugar in milk and dairy products. However, these statistics grossly exaggerate the incidence of true lactose intolerance. That's because testing for intolerance is based on studies which use a 50-gram test dose of lactose. A dose that size is the amount of lactose contained in one quart of milk! Indeed, most people will exhibit symptoms in a test using that concentrated a dose. There are only 12 grams of lactose in one cup (eight ounces) of milk and a mere 6 grams in a half cup. Just about everyone can handle that small an amount without any problem. The symptoms of lactose intolerance are abdominal cramps, bloating, gas, and diarrhea. These same symptoms can also signal other GI problems which may be unrelated to the consumption of dairy products. Careful testing is necessary to clarify the real cause.

What most people refer to as lactose intolerance is what researchers refer to as lactose maldigestion. People with lactose maldigestion may not have the same symptoms as those with intolerance, or may not have them to the same degree. Other factors may come into play: the time dairy products are consumed, what other foods are eaten at the same time, how much is eaten, and even cultural and psychological considerations.

True lactose intolerance can be temporary or permanent. Often it is brought on by gastric surgery, an intestinal infection, or some other intestinal problem. Antibiotics, some anti-inflammatory drugs, and other medications can affect lactose tolerance. In the truest sense, lactose intolerance is an upset caused by a shortage of the digestive enzyme lactase. Lactase, found on the surface of cells lining the small intestine, is necessary to digest milk and other dairy products. These foods contain the dietary sugar lactose. In early childhood, there is a natural decrease in the body's ability to produce lactase. That means that any lactose consumed has the *potential* to stay in the gut for a longer time and possibly cause gas, bloating, or diarrhea. Certain ethnic groups, including those of Asian and African descent, native Americans, and Jews, may have a problem digesting lactose. They are more likely to be lactose maldigesters, but not necessarily lactose intolerant. Chances are that they will not suffer GI problems when consuming milk and other dairy products in moderation, even though they are unable to fully digest lactose.

There is great variation in the way people handle different foods. The only way to discover *your* personal tolerance level is to consume small amounts of milk and other dairy products and make note of what happens. It is very likely that the problem is not as severe as you think.

What to Do about It

One test to detect true lactose intolerance involves drinking a large dose of lactose dissolved in water on an empty stomach and then measuring the rise in blood glucose. Even when this test is positive (indicating difficulty in processing lactose), smaller amounts of lactose may be tolerated. The complete exclusion of dairy products, therefore, may be unnecessary. It should be noted that for diabetics and people with malabsorption syndrome, the results of this test may be ambiguous. Similarly, people with delayed stomach emptying will probably have false-positive readings. Other tests are also available.

It is especially important for those who are definitely lactose intolerant to make wise food choices.

Yogurt and buttermilk are often tolerated by those who have been clinically diagnosed with this condition. Dairy products treated with a lactase preparation are often acceptable to the lactose intolerant as well. These include milk and cottage cheese sold under the brand names Lactaid® or DairyEase®. Soy milk and soy milk products do not contain lactose, so they are other possible options. Speak to a registered dietitian if you are truly lactose intolerant or if you think you are a maldigester. Be sure to discuss ways in which you can get an adequate amount of the nutrients. Remember that milk and dairy products provide 70 to 75 percent of the dietary calcium we consume. That's important for everyone at every age.

Those with maldigestion should try eating smaller amounts of milk or dairy products throughout the day. The Food Guide Pyramid recommendation for dairy products is just 2 servings a day for most adults and 3 servings for women who are pregnant or breastfeeding. By eating smaller portions, you can probably meet your quota with little or no effort. If you're worried about fat, there are lots of new low-fat and fat-free items from which to choose. Consume milk and dairy foods in combination with other foods and snacks to reduce any possible side effects. Eating pizza with cheese topping, skim milk with cereal, skim milk with graham crackers or a sandwich, casseroles made with milk and/or cheese, and homemade muffins or rice puddings made with milk will enable you to taper the effects of lactose maldigestion but still get important nutrients. Some individuals tolerate cocoa and chocolate milk better than regular milk. A little experimentation with foods such as these should help you to get your recommended servings each day. When you think about it, [2 or 3] that's not very much, especially when spread out over a few meals and snacks.

Jumping to the conclusion that you have a problem with lactose because a family member does isn't always correct. If you suspect you have a problem, make notes in your food diary regarding dairy products. Pay close attention to the amount and to the time of day you're eating these foods. Drinking a big glass of milk first thing in the morning or on an empty stomach late in the afternoon may cause distress for a lot of people, but does not necessarily indicate lactose intolerance. It is more likely to mean that you're a maldigester and could handle a smaller amount, perhaps with crackers or a piece of toast. These tips can help you put more nutritious foods back into your meals. An added bonus is that you'll enjoy those meals even more by doing so.

Wise Alternatives

Eliminating or reducing dairy products to fewer than 2 servings a day is not a good idea. If you've tried some of the previous suggestions without success, you still have

Be Good to Your Gut

some other possibilities to explore. To ensure a good intake of calcium and the other nutrients found in dairy products, try some of these suggestions.

Lactaid® Milk

This brand of milk is now sold in supermarkets throughout the country. It contains lactase and is available in low-fat and nonfat varieties, as well as in a version that is fortified with extra calcium. These milks tend to be a bit sweeter than regular milk. They can be used for drinking and in cooking. Lactaid® products break down almost 70 percent of the lactose, and few people are bothered by the remaining 30 percent. The latest Lactaid® milk product is 100 percent lactose-free.

Acidophilus Milk

Look in the dairy section for milk with a bacterium called lactobacillus acidophilus added to it. Some health food stores also carry acidophilus milk. What this product does is to increase bacterial count in the gut and ease the digestion of lactose.

Acidophilus milk tastes the same as regular milk, though some brands may vary. However, this milk can be used only for drinking, because heat destroys the beneficial bacteria. A few studies have shown that lactobacillus did not reduce the symptoms in lactose maldigesting subjects, so you may need to do a little personal testing to determine its effectiveness for you.

Lactase Enzyme Tablets and Drops

The lactase enzyme which you are lacking is available, usually in health-food stores or pharmacies, in liquid and tablet forms. A

Be Good to Your Gut

supply of these is especially useful when traveling. They can help you enjoy ice cream, cheeses, milk, casseroles, puddings, and other cooked foods that have dairy products as an ingredient. The tablets can be taken before or with a meal containing dairy products, while the drops can be added to milk 24 hours before consumption. Lactaid® is one of the brands to look for.

Cultured Milk Products and Cheese

Yogurt, sour cream, buttermilk, and some hard and soft-ripened cheeses have a reduced lactose content and do not cause gastric distress for lactose malabsorbers. Cured cheeses like Cheddar, aged Swiss, and Parmesan, along with sour cream, also have a reduced lactose content. The lactose in these products has been converted to lactic acid in the manufacturing process.

Yogurt with live-active cultures is usually the easiest for lactose-intolerant people to digest, because the lactose in it is already predigested. However, yogurt that has been heat-treated before fermentation will not have this benefit. Read the label to be sure. Dannon, for instance, adds lactobacillus acidophilus culture to many of its yogurts. That culture has the strongest ability to survive the acid environment in the stomach and produces an enzyme similar to intestinal lactase. The double benefit of that yogurt culture is that it reduces the amount of lactose in the yogurt and also helps the body digest the remaining lactose when the yogurt is eaten. Anyone who is lactose intolerant or a maldigester will need to experiment to find the amount of yogurt that is comfortable for them.

If you have been avoiding or eliminating dairy products, perhaps you can reconsider that decision. You may be pleasantly surprised to find that you can enjoy the flavor and good nutrition offered by this group of foods.

RESOURCES

This book is just one of many resources available to you. Once you've identified your particular problem, you can get more information from a variety of sources.

The following pages provide a brief national listing to get you started. In addition, the last page has some informative books which you may want to have on your bookshelf for handy reference.

Thumb through your local telephone directory as well. It might lead you to some convenient telephone numbers for assistance. Community hospitals and health maintenance organizations (HMOs) often have brochures and/or workshops that are helpful.

Good luck.

Organizations

American Association of Diabetes Educators
444 North Michigan Avenue
Suite 1240
Chicago, IL   60611-3901
800-TEAM-UP4 (832-6874)

Over 9,000 health professionals including dietitians, nurses, physicians, pharmacists, social workers, and exercise physiologists who specialize in diabetes education. A total of 100 chapters in the United States, including Alaska, Hawaii, and Puerto Rico. Consumers can call the toll-free number to get a referral for a certified diabetes educator in their local area.

American Institute of Hypnotherapy
16842 Von Karman Avenue
Suite 475
Irvine, CA 92714
714-261-6400

Publishes a directory of persons registered and certified to offer hypnotherapy; will also refer those seeking help to local contacts. The institute maintains a public information office for the general public, as well as a speakers' bureau which will provide lecturers to the public and interested parties. Books and self-hypnosis tapes are available by mail order.

Association for Applied Psychophysiology
and Biofeedback
10200 West 44th Street
Wheat Ridge, CO 80033

Send requests to above address with a self-addressed, stamped envelope.

Membership organization for over 1,800 professionals. Provides information and guidelines for consumers regarding biofeedback. The association will also provide a free listing of chapter contacts in areas around the country. A directory of members may be ordered for a separate fee.

Digestive Disease National Coalition
711 2nd Street, NE
Suite 200
Washington, DC 20002
202-544-7499

Informs the public and the health care community about digestive diseases; seeks federal funding for research, education, and training; and represents members' interests in federal and state legislation affecting digestive disease research, health care, and education. This organization also provides an informative brochure entitled When You Suffer the Pain and Discomfort of Digestive Diseases: Here's How We Can Help. The brochure lists organizations to contact for more information on a number of problems including heartburn, irritable bowel syndrome, and constipation.

International Foundation for Bowel
Dysfunction (IFBD)
P.O. Box 17864
Milwaukee, WI 53217
414-964-1799

Provides support and information for people affected by functional bowel disorders, including irritable bowel syndrome, constipation, diarrhea, pain, and incontinence. Publishes a quarterly newsletter called Participate as well as educational pamphlets and a fact sheet.

Intestinal Disease Foundation, Inc.
1323 Forbes Ave.
Suite 200
Pittsburgh, PA   15219
412-261-5888

Provides accurate, up-to-date medical information, patient education programs, support groups, a phone support network, and a quarterly newsletter entitled Intestinal Fortitude, for patients and their families living with intestinal diseases such as Crohn's disease, ulcerative colitis, Irritable Bowel Syndrome, diverticular disease, short gut syndrome, incontinence, and chronic diarrhea, gas, and constipation.

National Center for Nutrition and Dietetics (NCND)
The American Dietetic Association
216 W. Jackson Boulevard
Chicago, IL   60606-6995
Consumer Nutrition Hotline: 800-366-1655

Provides consumers with direct immediate access to reliable food and nutrition information. Callers may speak directly with a registered dietitian Monday through Friday, 10 AM to 5 PM, EST. Referrals to a dietitian in the caller's local area are available. In addition, callers may listen to regularly updated recorded nutrition messages in English and Spanish Monday through Friday, 9 AM to 9 PM, EST.

National Digestive Disease Information
Clearing House
2 Information Way
Bethesda, MD 20892-3570
Attn: BGG

The National Digestive Diseases Information Clearinghouse (NDDIC) is an information and referral service of the National Institute of Diabetes and Digestive and Kidney Diseases, one of the National Institutes of Health. The clearinghouse responds to written inquiries, develops and distributes publications about digestive diseases, and provides referrals to digestive disease organizations, including support groups. The NDDIC maintains a database of patient and professional education materials, from which literature searches are generated.

Food and Product Information

Bean Education & Awareness Network
115 Railway Plaza
Suite A108, Dept. PB
Scottsbluff, NE 69361
302 632-8239 (phone and fax)

Send a self-addressed, stamped business-sized envelope to receive a free brochure called It's Bean Healthy. Provides information on the role of beans in a healthy, high-fiber diet. Also includes several tasty, easy-to-prepare recipes.

The Dannon Company
P.O. Box 1102
Maple Plain, MN 55592
Mail requests only

The Dannon Information Center offers a booklet entitled You Asked About Lactobacillus Acidophilus as part of its nutrition and health series. This handy reference explains what cultures are and how they are used in making yogurt. Lactose intolerance information is also included. Send a legal-size, self-addressed, stamped envelope.

Nutrition Services Department
National Dairy Council
10255 West Higgins Road, Suite 900
Rosemont, IL 60463

An informative brochure on lactose intolerance, called Getting Along with Milk, is available to consumers. Please send 25 cents and a self-addressed stamped business-sized envelope marked "Getting Along with Milk" to the address listed above.

Supermarket Savvy Information & Resource Service
Leni Reed, MPH, RD
P.O. Box 666
Herndon, VA 22070-0666
703-742-3364

Newsletter called Supermarket Savvy. Six issues per year for health professionals, also available for consumers. Offers new product reviews and product-comparison charts. January and July issues feature the

236   *Be Good to Your Gut*

"Brand Name Shopping List," a comprehensive list of healthier foods by brand name.

Fitness and Exercise

The President's Council on Physical Fitness and Sports
Suite 250
701 Pennsylvania Avenue, NW
Washington, DC 20004

Offers information and publications on health and fitness. Pep Up Your Life, for mid-life and older adults, was developed in conjunction with the American Association of Retired Persons (AARP). Contains clear, easy-to-read information on nutrition and physical activity (primarily flexibility, strength, and endurance). It is free from the address above. In addition, The Nolan Ryan Fitness Guide offers handy information on developing an individual fitness program that includes aerobics, weight training, and stretching. There's also helpful information on caring for sports injuries. For a copy of the Nolan Ryan Fitness Guide, write to P.O. Box 22091, Albany, NY 12201-2091.

Walking Association
655 E. Rancho Catalina Place
Tuscon, AZ 85704
(520) 742-9589
Robert B. Sleight, Executive Director

Publishes newsletter, guides, and walking manuals; coordinates small walking groups; advises on walking benefits and techniques; consults on establishment of walking facilities.

For Your Bookshelf

The following books will provide helpful information. They are available in bookstores and in many libraries.

101 High Fiber Recipes. Corinne T. Netzer. Dell Publishing, 1992.

Doctor What Should I Eat? Isadore Rosenfeld, MD. Random House, 1995.

Gastrointestinal Health: A Self-Help Program. Steven Peikin, MD. Harper Collins, 1991.

The Grains Cookbook. Bert Greene. Workman Publishing, 1988.

Mayo Clinic Family Health Book: The Ultimate Home Medical Reference. David E. Larson, editor. William Morrow, 1990.

Total Nutrition: The Only Guide You'll Ever Need. Victor Herbert, MD, FACP, and Genell J. Subak-Sharpe, MS, editors. St. Martin's Press, 1995.

Your Gut Feelings: A Complete Guide to Living Better with Intestinal Problems. Henry D. Janowitz, MD. Oxford University Press, 1994.

The Wellness Book of IBS: How to Achieve Relief from Irritable Bowel Syndrome and Live a Symptom-Free Life. Deralee Scanlon, RD. St. Martin's Press, 1991.

REFERENCES

Robert Berkow, MD, editor. *The Merck Manual of Diagnosis and Therapy*, 16th edition. Merck & Co, 1992.

Sylvia Escott-Stump. *Nutrition and Diagnosis-Related Care.* 3rd edition. Lea & Febiger, 1992.

"The Heartburn Survey." The Gallup Organization, April 1995.

Victor Herbert, MD, editor. *Total Nutrition: The Only Guide You'll Ever Need.* St. Martin's Press, 1995.

L.K. Mahan and M. Arlin. *Krause's Food, Nutrition & Diet Therapy.* 8th edition. Saunders Publishing, 1992.

Jennifer Nelson, MS, RD, et al. *Mayo Clinic Diet Manual: A Handbook of Nutrition Practices*, 7th Edition. Mosby, 1994.

Steven Peckin, MD. *Gastrointestinal Health*. Harper Collins, 1991.

Isadore Rosenfeld, MD. *Doctor What Should I Eat?* Random House, 1995.

Deralee Scanlon, RD. *The Wellness Book of IBS.* St. Martin's Press, 1991.